STUDY GUIDE TO NEUROPSYCHIATRY AND CLINICAL NEUROSCIENCES

A Companion to
The American Psychiatric Publishing
Textbook of Neuropsychiatry and
Clinical Neurosciences, Fourth Edition

STUDY GUIDE TO NEUROPSYCHIATRY AND CLINICAL NEUROSCIENCES

A Companion to
The American Psychiatric Publishing
Textbook of Neuropsychiatry and
Clinical Neurosciences, Fourth Edition

James A. Bourgeois, O.D., M.D.

Associate Professor of Clinical Psychiatry and Allan Stoudemire Professor of
Psychosomatic Medicine, Department of Psychiatry and Behavioral Sciences
Director, Consultation-Liaison Service
University of California–Davis School of Medicine
Sacramento, California

Narriman C. Shahrokh

Chief Administrative Officer, Department of Psychiatry and Behavioral Sciences
University of California–Davis School of Medicine
Sacramento, California

Robert E. Hales, M.D., M.B.A.

Joe P. Tupin Professor and Chair, Department of Psychiatry and Behavioral Sciences
University of California–Davis School of Medicine
Director, UC Davis Health System Behavioral Health Center
Director, UC Davis Sierra Health Foundation MD/MBA Fellowship Program
Medical Director, Mental Health Services, County of Sacramento
Sacramento, California

Stuart C. Yudofsky, M.D.

D. C. and Irene Ellwood Professor and Chair, Menninger Department of Psychiatry
and Behavioral Sciences, Baylor College of Medicine
Chief, Psychiatry Service, The Methodist Hospital
Houston, Texas

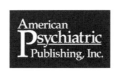

American Psychiatric Publishing, Inc.

Washington, DC
London, England

Copyright © 2006 American Psychiatric Publishing, Inc.

ALL RIGHTS RESERVED

Manufactured in the United States of America on acid-free paper
10   09   08   07   06   5   4   3   2   1

ISBN   1-58562-259-1
ISBN-13   978-1-58562-259-7

First Edition

Typeset in Revival BT and Adobe's The Mix

American Psychiatric Publishing, Inc.
1000 Wilson Boulevard
Arlington, VA 22209-3901
www.appi.org

Contents

Answer Guide

Page numbers in the Answer Guide refer to

The American Psychiatric Publishing Textbook of

Neuropsychiatry and Clinical Neurosciences, Fourth Edition.

Visit **www.appi.org** for more information about this textbook.

| | | |

Purchase the online version of this Study Guide at

www.cme.psychiatryonline.org

and receive instant scoring and CME credits.

C H A P T E R   1

Cellular and Molecular Biology of the Neuron

Select the single best response for each question.

1.1 In the central nervous system (CNS), both chemical and electrical synapses are critical for neural activity. Regarding chemically mediated synapses and their neurotransmitters, which of the following is true?

A. Chemical synapses are faster than electrical synapses.
B. Chemical synapses are limited in utility because they do not allow for signal amplification.
C. Chemical synapses can modulate the activity of other cells through activation of second-messenger cascades.
D. Small molecule transmitters (e.g., glutamate, γ-aminobutyric acid [GABA], and glycine) are stored in large, dense-core vesicles.
E. Neuropeptides (e.g., somatostatin, endorphins, and enkephalins) mediate fast synaptic transmission.

1.2 GABA receptors are ubiquitous in the CNS and have different conformational and neurophysiological properties. Regarding these receptors, which of the following is true?

A. $GABA_A$ receptors are metabotropic receptors.
B. The $GABA_A$ receptor-channel complex is composed of five subunits.
C. $GABA_B$ receptors are primarily located postsynaptically.
D. Clinical actions of benzodiazepines and barbiturates are proportional to their binding potential at $GABA_B$ receptors.
E. Benzodiazepines increase GABA current by increasing the amount of "open" time in receptor channels.

1.3 The generation of long-term potentiation (LTP) is critical in the neurophysiology of memory. In the mechanism of the generation of LTP in the mammalian hippocampus, which of the following is true?

A. LTP results from the coincident activation of α-amino-3-hydroxy-5-methylisoxazole-4-propionic acid (AMPA) receptors and postsynaptic hyperpolarization.
B. LTP requires Ca^{2+} efflux from postsynaptic neurons.
C. "Silent" synapses contain only AMPA receptors before induction of LTP and can be activated by insertion of new *N*-methyl-D-aspartate (NMDA) receptors.
D. LTP is composed of early and late phases, both of which require induction of new protein synthesis.
E. LTP and long-term depression (LTD) function in a dynamic equilibrium to maintain memory.

1.4   In neuronal development and modulation, the neuron develops following a specific sequence of steps. Which of the following is the correct order for neuronal growth?

    A. Determination, proliferation, migration, axonal elongation, synapse formation, synapse refinement, cell death.

    B. Determination, migration, proliferation, axonal elongation, synapse formation, synapse refinement, cell death.

    C. Determination, axonal elongation, proliferation, migration, synapse formation, synapse refinement, cell death.

    D. Proliferation, determination, migration, axonal elongation, synapse formation, synapse refinement, cell death.

    E. Proliferation, determination, axonal elongation, migration, synapse refinement, synapse formation, cell death.

1.5   In neuronal migration, neurons migrate from the "inside out" to reach their final spatial destinations within a laminar structure. What is the laminar organization of neuronal zones, from pial surface to the ventricles?

    A. Marginal zone, cortical plate, subplate, intermediate zone, subventricular zone, ventricular zone.

    B. Marginal zone, cortical plate, subplate, intermediate zone, ventricular zone, subventricular zone.

    C. Cortical plate, subplate, marginal zone, intermediate zone, subventricular zone, ventricular zone.

    D. Cortical plate, marginal zone, subplate, intermediate zone, ventricular zone, subventricular zone.

    E. Marginal zone, cortical plate, subplate, ventricular zone, intermediate zone, subventricular zone.

1.6   In the stages of neuronal maturation, the final stage is often apoptosis. The process of apoptosis is characterized by all of the following properties *except*

    A. It is a genetically programmed form of cell death.

    B. It occurs to cells deprived of neurotrophic fibers.

    C. Cytoplasmic shrinkage occurs.

    D. Ribonucleic acid (RNA) and protein synthesis is required for this process.

    E. An inflammatory response is triggered.

1.7   Several clinical neuropsychiatric disorders can be linked to specific neuroanatomic loci and/or particular neuropathological processes. Regarding the neuropathology of various neuropsychiatric disorders, which of the following is true?

    A. Striatal degeneration in Huntington's disease is linked to underproduction of a critical synaptic vesicle–associated protein.

    B. A delayed result of a viral infection may be causative in some cases of Parkinson's disease.

    C. 1-Methyl-4-phenyl-1,2,3,6-tetrahydropyridine (MPTP) may produce Parkinson's disease by receptor occupancy and blockade, rather than a neurotoxic mechanism.

    D. Parkinson's disease may also be caused by pathological excess of neurotrophic factors.

    E. Alzheimer's disease features loss of basal forebrain cholinergic neurons, which may follow an excess of or aberrant handling of nerve growth factor.

CHAPTER 2

Human Electrophysiology and Basic Sleep Mechanisms

Select the single best response for each question.

2.1   The electroencephalogram (EEG) features tracings of brain activity that are classified in frequency bands, which correlate with different central nervous system (CNS) actions. Which of the following is true regarding EEG frequency bands?

   A.   Delta waves (4–8 Hz) are associated with rapid eye movement (REM) sleep.
   B.   Alpha waves (8–14 Hz) are best recorded over the parietal region.
   C.   Alpha rhythm occurs during wakefulness, generally appearing on eye closure and vanishing on eye opening.
   D.   The genesis of alpha rhythms has been established to be in the thalamus.
   E.   Beta and gamma bands occur over nonoverlapping frequency ranges greater than 14 Hz.

2.2   Sleep is characterized by a sequence of sleep stages with specific EEG and behavioral correlates. In sleep studies, which of the following is true?

   A.   The typical polysomnogram consists of simultaneous monitoring of the EEG, electromyogram (EMG), and electro-oculogram (EOG).
   B.   Stage I sleep is characterized by the emergence of 14–16 Hz sleep spindles.
   C.   Stages III and IV sleep feature (respectively) greater and lesser occurrence of 0.5–4 Hz delta waves.
   D.   As the sleep period progresses, the subject spends less time in REM sleep with successive sleep cycles.
   E.   It is more difficult to arouse a subject from REM sleep than from Stage IV sleep.

2.3   Sleep patterns (both on EEG and in sleep behavior) change predictably across the life span. Regarding the change in sleep architecture over time, which of the following is true?

   A.   Infants sleep one-half of the time, with REM sleep occupying one-half of total sleep time.
   B.   The percentage of REM sleep declines rapidly throughout childhood, and the adult percentage of REM sleep is reached by age 20 years.
   C.   Adults spend approximately 35% of total sleep time in REM.
   D.   Non-REM (NREM) sleep (Stages III and IV) is minimal in newborns.
   E.   NREM sleep reaches a maximum by age 20 years before subsequently declining.

2.4   CNS activity as recorded by the EEG has been localized to various arousal mechanisms. Regarding the neurophysiology of EEG activation, which of the following is true?

   A. Brainstem cholinergic nuclei (laterodorsal and pedunculopontine tegmental nuclei, LDT/PPT) have high discharge rates only in waking, with low discharge rates in REM and slow-wave sleep (SWS).
   B. EEG synchronization refers to the EEG of wakefulness.
   C. Brainstem reticular neuronal projections, using inhibitory amino acid neurotransmission, also participate in EEG activation.
   D. Locus coeruleus and dorsal raphe nucleus monoaminergic neurons are active in REM sleep.
   E. Projections from the basal forebrain nucleus basalis of Meynert play an important role in EEG activation.

2.5   Adenosine has been demonstrated to have specific roles in sleep physiology. Regarding the role of adenosine in sleep, which of the following is true?

   A. Adenosine's role mediating sleepiness following prolonged wakefulness appears to be mediated by excitation of basal forebrain neurons.
   B. Stimulant beverages (e.g., coffee, tea) increase alertness by an agonist effect on adenosine receptors.
   C. Increased metabolism leads to an increase in extracellular adenosine in the basal forebrain.
   D. Basal forebrain extracellular adenosine levels decrease with prolonged wakefulness.
   E. With prolonged wakefulness, adenosine levels change uniformly in various brain regions important to behavioral state control.

2.6   Acetylcholine has been found to have important roles in sleep structure. Regarding cholinergic mechanisms in REM sleep, which of the following is true?

   A. Injection of acetylcholine agonists into the pontine reticular formation produces a REM-like state by activation of primarily nicotinic receptors.
   B. Approximately 50% of reticular formation neurons are excited by cholinergic agonists, primarily via nicotinic receptor effects.
   C. Cholinergic neurons are critical in the production of the low-voltage, fast EEG pattern in REM sleep and upon awakening.
   D. Electrical stimulation of the LDT decreases REM sleep.
   E. Cholinergic neurons may be critical in producing hyperpolarization of reticular effector neurons for REM sleep events.

2.7   Narcolepsy is a sleep disorder that causes significant disruption in patients' lives. Regarding narcolepsy, all of the following are true *except*

   A. It is a chronic sleep disorder.
   B. Patients experience excessive daytime sleepiness.
   C. Recent research shows undetectable levels of the neuropeptide orexin in narcolepsy patients.
   D. Delayed onset of REM is typical.
   E. Hypnagogic hallucinations are common.

CHAPTER 3

Functional Neuroanatomy: Neuropsychological Correlates of Cortical and Subcortical Damage

Select the single best response for each question.

3.1   Cortical localization of specific functions can be conceptualized on both a "right-left" dichotomy and an "anterior-posterior" one. Regarding lateral and longitudinal specialization of cortical functions, which of the following statements is true?

A. Less than 50% of left-handed persons are left-brain dominant for language functions.
B. Whereas the majority of the population process spoken and written language with the left hemisphere, languages derived from visuogestural signals (e.g., American Sign Language) are primarily processed in the right hemisphere.
C. In most subjects, the right hemisphere processes nonverbal information, such as complex visual patterns and nonverbal auditory information.
D. Posterior regions of the brain are primarily responsible for the execution of motor behavior.
E. Prosodic expression is a right-hemisphere function localized in the anatomical counterpart to Wernicke's area in the left hemisphere.

3.2   The hippocampal complex is a critical structure of the mesial temporal region of the temporal lobes. Which of the following statements about the hippocampal complex (structure and/or function) is true?

A. Anatomically, the hippocampal complex includes the hippocampus and amygdala.
B. The left hippocampal complex subserves the acquisition of new verbal material, and the right hippocampal complex is responsible for the acquisition of novel nonverbal material.
C. The hippocampal complexes are equally responsible for the acquisition of declarative and nondeclarative memory.
D. Patients with Alzheimer's disease with hippocampal damage exhibit marked impairment of both anterograde memory and the learning of novel perceptuomotor skills.
E. The hippocampal complex is a principal storage repository for "old" memories.

3.3 Perceptual and communication functions involve several complementary cortical functions, all of which must be integrated for normal perception of the environment and use of language. Regarding the functions of lexical retrieval ("naming") and visual recognition, which of the following statements is true?

A. Lexical retrieval is localized in the inferotemporal region of the temporal lobe, sparing the temporal pole.

B. Lesions in the temporal lobe that impair lexical retrieval typically impair other language functions such as grammar, syntax, and repetition.

C. Damage to the right anterolateral temporal region has been reported to cause a defect in naming of facial expressions.

D. The occipitotemporal junction consists of the posterior part of the inferotemporal region plus the superior portions of Brodmann's areas 17, 18, and 19.

E. Prosopagnosia, the inability to recognize previously known faces, is usually accompanied by an inability to recognize gender and age from face information.

3.4 Balint's syndrome is a devastating "central" disorder of visually related behaviors. Which of the following is true regarding Balint's syndrome?

A. It is caused by a lesion of the ventral component of the occipital cortex.

B. The lesion affects the primary visual cortex but spares the visual association cortices.

C. Balint's syndrome can only be produced with bilateral occipital lesions.

D. The three cardinal clinical features are visual disorientation, ocular apraxia, and optic ataxia.

E. Ocular apraxia refers to a disturbance in visually guided reaching behavior (e.g., accurately pointing at a target object using visual guidance).

3.5 The occipital lobes are exclusively devoted to processing visual information. Regarding the neuropsychological consequences of various occipital lesions, which of the following is true?

A. Acquired achromatopsia involves variable parts of the visual field and is typically associated with impairment in form vision.

B. Acquired achromatopsia is associated with impairment in the naming of colors.

C. A patient with a unilateral left occipitotemporal lesion may have right hemiachromatopsia but will rarely have an associated alexia.

D. Patients with apperceptive visual agnosia will have difficulty in producing the image of a whole entity when given just a part of a visual stimulus (e.g., they cannot imagine a car as the source of a wheel when presented with the image of a wheel).

E. Patients with pure alexia cannot read whole sentences but can always read single words or letters.

3.6   The parietal lobes are crucial for language, mathematical, and recognition functions. Regarding neuropsychological deficits from parietal lobe lesions, which of the following is true?

A. Wernicke's aphasia is characterized by fluent paraphasic speech and defective aural comprehension but preserved simple repetition.
B. Conduction aphasia is associated with profoundly defective verbatim repetition, nonfluent speech, and impaired reading comprehension.
C. Lesions to the inferior parietal lobule may lead to acalculia, an acquired inability to perform simple mathematical calculations.
D. Neglect syndromes from right-sided inferior parietal lobule lesions are confined to neglect of intrapersonal space.
E. Anosognosia refers to the patient's lack of concern with (rather than lack of recognition of) a neurological and/or neuropsychological deficit.

3.7   The frontal lobes are responsible for a wide array of behaviors, ranging from simple interpersonal communication to memory to interpersonal conduct. Which of the following statements is true regarding the neuropsychological correlates of frontal lobe dysfunction?

A. Akinetic mutism may follow lesions to the superior mesial aspect of the frontal lobe.
B. The patient with akinetic mutism makes no effort to communicate by any modality and will not track moving targets with smooth pursuit eye movements.
C. Akinetic mutism is typically more severe with right- as opposed to left-sided lesions.
D. Lesions to the basal forebrain may cause an amnestic syndrome characterized by an absence of confabulation.
E. Lesions to the ventromedial frontal lobe may cause the condition of acquired sociopathy, which is typically associated with an amnestic syndrome and diffuse conventional neuropsychological deficits.

C H A P T E R   4

Nervous, Endocrine, and Immune System Interactions in Psychiatry

Select the single best response for each question.

4.1   The immune system is characterized by a complex series of cells, proteins, and functional systems. Regarding the basic organization of the immune system, which of the following is true?

    A. All immune cells are derived from hematopoietic stem cells, which are located both in the bone marrow and in the peripheral circulation.

    B. The two developmental pathways for stem cells are the myeloid line (leading to B cells, T cells, and natural killer [NK] cells) and the lymphoid line (leading to monocytes and granulocytes).

    C. Cytokines are soluble immune signaling factors solely responsible for the regulation of cell movement.

    D. "Proinflammatory cytokines" include interleukin (IL)-1, interleukin-6, and tumor necrosis factor-alpha and are produced primarily by mast cells

    E. Type I interferons (IFNs), IFN-α and IFN-β, have both immunostimulatory and antiproliferative effects.

4.2   Natural and acquired immunity serve complementary functions through different mechanisms. Regarding the mechanisms and immunological roles of natural and acquired immunity, which of the following statements is true?

    A. Innate, or "natural" immunity is primarily mediated by phagocytes (e.g., monocytes and basophils) and NK cells.

    B. The acute phase response involves the production of acute phase reactants by the peripheral tissues to isolate invading pathogens.

    C. The complement system, acting through a cascade of proteins, is an important part of acquired immunity.

    D. The four sequential phases of acquired immunity are induction, activation, effector, and memory.

    E. T cell–mediated immunity is referred to as humoral immunity because this immunity can be transferred by cell-free blood products.

4.3   Stress and immune response have been examined in human subjects in several naturalistic settings. Which of the following statements is true?

A. Elderly caregivers of spouses with Alzheimer's disease have been shown to exhibit decreased lymphocyte proliferation and IL-2 production and a decreased ratio of T-suppressor to T-helper cells.

B. Immunologic effects of long-term stress have included decreased white blood cells, increased peripheral blood lymphocytes, and a decreased ratio of T-helper to T-suppressor cells.

C. In long-term naturalistic stressor studies, nonsocial stressors tend to have a greater immunological effect than social stressors.

D. Spousal caregivers of dementia patients have been found to have impaired wound healing when compared with matched control subjects.

E. Medical students facing examinations and spousal caregivers of Alzheimer's disease patients have been found to have decreased antibody responses to hepatitis A and influenza vaccines.

4.4   The relationship between cancer and psychological stressors has been examined. Which of the following is true?

A. A large Danish study found an increase in cancer, allergic disease, and autoimmune disease in parents whose child was diagnosed with cancer.

B. Major depression has been consistently found to increase the risk of a subsequent new diagnosis of cancer.

C. Research data suggests that psychological variables have a greater impact on the *course* of cancer rather than dramatically increasing its *incidence* risk.

D. Studies of clinical psychiatric interventions in cancer patients (e.g., cognitive-behavioral therapy and group therapy) have consistently found an increase in cancer longevity for patients receiving psychiatric treatments.

E. Studies of psychiatric interventions for cancer patients have generally been targeted to patients at higher risk for psychiatric illness.

4.5   Immune function has been studied in patients with depression. Which of the following is true?

A. Peripheral blood findings in depressed patients have included increased lymphocytes, decreased neutrophils, and decreased NK cell activity.

B. A syndrome of "sickness behavior" mimicking major depression follows administration of IFN-α and IL-2.

C. Cerebrospinal fluid (CSF) studies of depressed patients have demonstrated increased levels of IL-6 and soluble IL-6 receptors and decreased levels of IL-1-β.

D. Female patients with depression are more likely to exhibit NK cell decreases than male patients.

E. Decreased acute phase proteins have been found in depressed patients.

4.6   Immunologic function in schizophrenia has revealed which one of the following?

A. Peripheral blood findings in schizophrenic patients include decreased B cells, CD4+ lymphocytes, and monocytes.

B. Decreased acute phase proteins have been reported.

C. Increased CD5+ cells have been found, suggesting an autoimmune mechanism in schizophrenia.

D. CSF findings in schizophrenic patients include decreased IL-2 and soluble IL-6 receptors.

E. Increased IL-2 levels in schizophrenia are specific for an autoimmune, rather than infectious, mechanism in the genesis of schizophrenia.

CHAPTER 5

Bedside Neuropsychiatry: Eliciting the Clinical Phenomena of Neuropsychiatric Illness

Select the single best response for each question.

5.1 The clinical examination of the neuropsychiatric patient involves thorough data gathering and specific interviewing strategies. Which of the following statements is true regarding the history and/or examination of a neuropsychiatric patient?

A. When questioning a head-injured patient, the duration of loss of consciousness or coma is considered the best indicator for severity of traumatic brain injury.

B. Assessment of the length of posttraumatic amnesia should be discerned only by questioning the patient because hospital records are generally unreliable.

C. A loss of capacity for divided attention is more suggestive of "functional" psychiatric illness than cerebral disease or injury.

D. Regarding observations of dream activity in traumatic brain injury, loss of dream material is specific for left, rather than right, parietal lobe injury.

E. Abnormal oral/feeding behavior, such as mouthing and consumption of nonfood items suggests Klüver-Bucy syndrome (bilateral amygdalar disease).

5.2 Minor physical anomalies may offer a clue to the interpretation of neuropsychiatric syndromes. Regarding the content and application of the Waldrop scale of minor physical anomalies as pertains to neuropsychiatry, which of the following is true?

A. The items on this scale are limited to abnormalities of the head and neck.

B. Minor physical abnormalities specified are not found in normal individuals and reliably identify neuropsychiatric illness.

C. Deviant physical development of the head occurs from the fourth to sixth months of fetal life.

D. Minor physical anomalies are associated with schizophrenia, including late-onset schizophrenia.

E. Dysmorphic features can readily classify the type of syndrome responsible for mental retardation.

5.3   Assessment of eye movements may assist neuropsychiatric diagnosis. Regarding eye movements in neuropsychiatry, which of the following is true?

A. It is generally advisable for the clinician to make inferential descriptions ("Patient was looking at source of hallucinated voices") rather than phenomenological descriptions ("Patient suddenly looked to his left several times in mid-sentence").
B. Stevens's studies and subsequent laboratory studies of eye movement disorders in schizophrenia have addressed saccadic movements.
C. Failure of voluntary lateral gaze is a hallmark of progressive supranuclear palsy.
D. Visual grasping refers to the inability to suppress reflex saccadic eye movements and is seen in schizophrenia.
E. Eye movement disorders, such as slowed saccades and an inability to make a saccadic eye movement without simultaneous head movements, are uncommon in Huntington's disease.

5.4   Speech disorders are relatively common in neuropsychiatric illness. Regarding clinical abnormalities of speech, which of the following is true?

A. In pseudobulbar palsy, slow, strained, and slurred speech are only infrequently accompanied by dysphagia, drooling, and disturbed emotional expression.
B. Acquired stuttering may follow stroke, psychotropic drug ingestion, and extrapyramidal disease.
C. Developmental and acquired stuttering are both characterized by involuntary movements of the face and head, reminiscent of dystonias.
D. Aprosodia (the emotional analog of aphasia) is produced solely by right-sided hemispheric lesions.
E. Echolalia refers to a simple "parroting back" of the examiner's speech by the patient, with no modifications of content or grammar.

5.5   The movement disorders in Huntington's disease and tardive dyskinesia can appear to overlap in some patients. Which of the following movement types is more common in Huntington's disease rather than in tardive dyskinesia?

A. Repetitive stereotypic movements.
B. Oro-buccal-lingual site abnormal movements.
C. Improvement of facial dyskinesias with tongue protrusion.
D. Postural instability.
E. Marching in place.

5.6   Various reflexes can be elicited in the neuropsychiatric patient. Regarding the use of primitive reflexes in clinical examination, which of the following is true?

A. All primitive reflexes reflect underlying neuropathology.
B. The grasp, snout, and palmomental reflexes can be elicited with careful examination in the majority of schizophrenia patients.
C. Primitive reflexes in demented patients predict more cognitive impairment for a given level of functional impairment but do not predict prognosis.
D. They are more common in vascular dementia localized in the frontal lobe than in frontotemporal dementia.
E. The grasp reflex is associated with dysfunction of the supplementary motor area.

5.7 Orientation and memory are basic parts of the clinical examination of the neuropsychiatric patient. Regarding tests of orientation and memory, which of the following is true?

A. The majority of delirium patients are disoriented for person, place, and time.
B. The delirium patient mistakes the "familiar for the unfamiliar," whereas the schizophrenic patient mistakes the "unfamiliar for the familiar."
C. In attention testing, the insertion of a single number in "forward" order in the backward counting test ("20, 19, 18, 17, 18") is rarely significant.
D. Neglect following a right-hemisphere stroke is usually a permanent deficit.
E. Improved recall with semantic cueing is common in frontal-subcortical dementia.

5.8 Thought disorders in the neuropsychiatric patient are best distinguished as disorders of form and content. In assessment of disorders of form and content of thought in the neuropsychiatric patient, which of the following is true?

A. Confabulation, the fabrication of false "factual" material by the patient, may be either spontaneous or in response to physician inquiries and is exclusively seen in amnestic disorders.
B. The Ganser state, or *Vorbeireden (Vorbeigehen)*, is a syndrome of approximate answers that is caused by a focal cerebral lesion.
C. The Charles Bonnet syndrome is characterized by visual hallucinations without other neuropsychiatric findings and is often accompanied by visual deficits.
D. Vividly colored but unformed visual hallucinations are typical with disease of the upper brainstem and/or thalamus.
E. Pathological laughter and crying are discordant with the enduring emotional state but are only elicited by an emotion-laden stimulus such as seeing strong affective expression in another person.

CHAPTER 6

Electrodiagnostic Techniques in Neuropsychiatry

Select the single best response for each question.

6.1 The electroencephalogram (EEG) may be a valuable diagnostic test in neuropsychiatry, particularly in enigmatic cases or obscure clinical presentations. Which of the following statements is true?

A. The EEG itself is likely to lead to a precise diagnosis in the majority of cases because of highly specific abnormalities on surface electrode tracings.

B. Disorders affecting deep brain structures or characterized by slow, indolent neuronal damage will typically affect electroencephalographic tracings.

C. Delirium is associated with generalized slowing and irregular high-voltage beta activity.

D. Dementia is associated with paroxysmal bifrontal delta activity and asymmetry between cerebral hemispheres.

E. Benzodiazepine intoxication features characteristic background slowing with the superimposition of alpha, but not beta, frequencies.

6.2 The P300 potential may be affected by certain neuropsychiatric illnesses. Which of the following is true?

A. Schizophrenic patients typically have increased P300 amplitude.

B. Abnormal P300 potentials in schizophrenia are specific to medication-naive patients, because antipsychotic medication normalizes the P300 potentials in patients with schizophrenia.

C. Among personality-disordered patients, borderline personality disorder has been found to have more P300 potential abnormalities.

D. Prolonged P300 latency, a common finding in normal aging, is blunted in schizophrenia.

E. P300 potential abnormalities in schizophrenia appear to be unrelated to cognitive deficits.

6.3 The EEG is most specific for evaluation of seizure disorders. Which of the following is true?

A. Epilepsy has a prevalence in the general population of approximately 0.5%.

B. "Spikes" and "sharp waves" in the electroencephalographic tracings of epileptic patients are rarely associated with "polyspikes" and rarely followed by slow waves.

C. Interictal electroencephalographic abnormalities are rare in epilepsy.

D. "Epileptiform" activity on EEG is present in 25%–30% of the normal population.

E. Epileptiform electroencephalographic tracings are relatively common in schizophrenia but much less so in major depression with psychotic features.

6.4   The EEG may reveal abnormalities in the cognitive disorders as well as in normal senescence. Which of the following is true?

   A. Background alpha rhythm diminishes steadily between young adulthood and old age.
   B. Low-voltage beta activity increases steadily throughout life unless there is the emergence of dementia.
   C. Mild diffuse slowing is found in the majority of patients over age 75 years.
   D. Electroencephalographic slowing has been correlated with cognitive impairment in dementia but is not related to the number of senile plaques seen neuropathologically.
   E. Patients with histologically proven Alzheimer's disease have a nearly 100% risk of abnormal EEG.

6.5   Schizophrenia has been studied with regard to associated electroencephalographic anomalies. Which of the following statements is true regarding the EEG and schizophrenia?

   A. Although electroencephalographic abnormalities in schizophrenia are more common than in normal healthy subjects, a characteristic "schizophrenic EEG" has not been described.
   B. Numerous studies with adequate control subjects have consistently shown a rate of 80% for abnormal EEG in schizophrenia.
   C. Schizophrenic patients have a greatly increased risk of seizure disorder, likely correlating with their greater risk of abnormal EEGs.
   D. When electroencephalographic hemispheric asymmetries have been seen in schizophrenic patients, the right hemisphere is generally implicated.
   E. A strong family history of schizophrenia predicts an abnormal EEG in a schizophrenic patient.

C H A P T E R 7

The Neuropsychological Evaluation

Select the single best response for each question.

7.1   A patient tells you that she has an IQ score at the 98th percentile. This corresponds to a *z* score of

   A. −2.0.
   B. +2.0.
   C. +3.0.
   D. +4.0.
   E. 98.

7.2   A test has validity when

   A. It measures what it purports to measure.
   B. It is given to the same individual at different times and the scores are consistent.
   C. It was constructed with a large normative sample.
   D. It is sensitive to brain damage.
   E. It has high specificity.

7.3   Neuropsychological examinations include multiple measures of many cognitive functions. Multiple measures, which involve similar or related abilities, increase the _____ of findings.

   A. Specificity.
   B. Variability.
   C. Validity.
   D. Quality.
   E. Reliability.

7.4   There is a tendency for left hemisphere lesions to produce a relatively depressed _____ in a neuropsychological test battery.

   A. Full-scale IQ.
   B. Performance IQ.
   C. Verbal IQ.
   D. Rey Complex Figure.
   E. Grooved Pegboard Test score.

7.5   The ability to hold information in mind while performing a mental task is called

    A. Processing speed.
    B. Visual acuity.
    C. Sensitivity.
    D. Working memory.
    E. Specificity.

7.6   The abilities involved in formulating goals, planning, effectively carrying out goal-directed plans, monitoring, and self-correcting are collectively called

    A. Executive functions.
    B. Motor functions.
    C. Perception.
    D. Praxis.
    E. Constructional ability.

7.7   The L, F, and K scales of the Minnesota Multiphasic Personality Inventory (MMPI) and MMPI-2 are also called the _____ scales.

    A. Reliability.
    B. Validity.
    C. Neurological.
    D. Compliant.
    E. Symptom.

7.8   The most popular neuropsychological test battery in the United States is the

    A. Category test.
    B. Luria-Nebraska Neuropsychological Battery.
    C. Halstead-Reitan Battery.
    D. Dementia Rating Scale.
    E. Mini-Mental State Exam.

C H A P T E R 8

Clinical Imaging in Neuropsychiatry

Select the single best response for each question.

8.1 The role of neuroimaging in neuropsychiatry has been evolving and in some areas remains controversial. In recent years, technical improvements have led to a broader use of neuroimaging. Which of the following would *not* be an indication for neuroimaging?

A. Cognitive decline verging on a diagnosis of dementia.
B. Traumatic brain injury.
C. Initial presentation of psychotic illness, regardless of age of patient.
D. New onset of nonpsychotic major depression in a 40-year-old patient.
E. Psychiatric symptoms in an alcohol-dependent patient.

8.2 The clinical benefit of neuroimaging can be increased by the judicious use of contrast agents. Which of the following statements about contrast-enhanced computed tomography (CT) is *not* true?

A. Contrast agents do not penetrate the intact blood-brain barrier (BBB).
B. Contrast agents may be visualized in the parenchyma of the brain in autoimmune disease, central nervous system infections, and tumors because of disruption of the BBB.
C. Vascular anomalies, such as arteriovenous malformations and aneurysms, can be visualized more readily by contrast-enhanced scans despite preservation of the BBB.
D. Xenon-enhanced CT (Xe/CT) may enhance identification of structural anomalies on CT, but cannot be repeated frequently and adds substantial expense.
E. Despite their greater expense, nonionic contrast agents are preferred because of their much lower risk of allergic reactions.

8.3 The advent of magnetic resonance imaging (MRI) has significantly added to the anatomical detail that can be obtained by clinical neuroimaging. Although the procedure is safe for the vast majority of patients, there are some specific safety concerns that may limit its use. Which of the following is *not* true?

A. Cardiac pacemakers may be damaged by the magnetic field, which can alter programming and increase the risk of arrhythmias.
B. Pacemaker wires can develop dangerous levels of electrical current, leading to burns and/or movement of the wires and pacemaker.
C. Other implanted devices, such as cochlear implants, dental implants, and bone-growth stimulators, can be demagnetized or be moved by MRI.
D. Continuous physiological monitoring of a patient during an MRI procedure is not possible.
E. Caution is needed before subjecting a pregnant patient to an MRI.

8.4 The neuropsychiatrist must frequently choose among various structural neuroimaging protocols for patient evaluation. In this decision, the clinician should keep in mind that CT and MRI are each preferred for imaging of certain neuropsychiatric conditions. Which of the following conditions is better evaluated by MRI, as opposed to CT?

A. Acute cerebral hemorrhage with delirium.
B. Subcortical dementia from Parkinson's disease.
C. Calcified lesions from tuberous sclerosis.
D. Traumatic brain injury with physical evidence of skull fracture.
E. Acute psychosis without focal neurological signs when a "screening" examination is desired.

8.5 The caudate nucleus is the site of focal degeneration in Huntington's disease. The caudate nucleus, together with the putamen, receives projection inputs from numerous other areas of the brain and also has several outflow tracts. As such, this system can be regarded as having significant "relay" functions. Because of the complexity of these connections, many distinct neuropsychiatric symptoms may follow damage to the caudate nucleus. Which of the following is *not* a commonly reported deficit of caudate nucleus dysfunction?

A. Mania without episodes of depression.
B. Behavioral disinhibition.
C. Disorganization.
D. Aphasia.
E. Personality changes.

8.6 The substantia nigra is composed of the pars reticulata and pars compacta. Which of the following is true regarding the substantia nigra and neuropsychiatric symptoms attributed to lesions of this area?

A. The pars reticulata has dopaminergic projections to the caudate nucleus and putamen.
B. The pars compacta sends efferents to the thalamus and subthalamus.
C. Lesions to the substantia nigra produce primarily cognitive, rather than behavioral, symptoms.
D. Mania is more common than depression with substantia nigra lesions.
E. Apraxia, ataxia, and aggressive behavior are common with substantia nigra lesions.

8.7 The amygdala and thalamus have important anatomical connections and participate intimately in the regulation of emotion, behavior, and memory. Which of the following is true?

A. Lesions localized to the amygdala typically result in memory, rather than behavioral or emotional, symptoms.
B. Patients with amygdalar lesions will often present with diminished appetites for sexual behavior and feeding behavior.
C. Damage to the left medial thalamus produces deficits in visual memory.
D. Bilateral damage to the thalamus may result in either thalamic amnesia or dementia.
E. Disturbances in autonomic functions, mood, and circadian rhythm may be caused by lesions of the anterior, but not medial, thalamus.

C H A P T E R 9

Functional Neuroimaging in Psychiatry

Select the single best response for each question.

9.1   There are several different approaches to functional neuroimaging. Which of the following is *not* true?

   A. Positron emission tomography (PET) and single photon emission computed tomography (SPECT) both use radioactivity to measure brain metabolism, cerebral blood flow, and neurotransmitter receptors, but PET is more widely available.
   B. Functional magnetic resonance imaging (fMRI) employs levels of blood oxygenation to estimate neural activation.
   C. Arterial spin tagging is used to estimate cerebral blood flow.
   D. Magnetic resonance spectroscopy (MRS) assesses local chemical concentrations.
   E. Magnetoencephalography (MEG) assesses magnetic fluctuations associated with regional brain activity.

9.2   Regarding PET, which of the following is true?

   A. The most commonly used radioisotopes in PET are oxygen 15 (^{15}O) water for imaging of metabolism and fluorine 18 (^{18}F) fluorodeoxyglucose (FDG) to image cerebral blood flow.
   B. PET can be used to image neurotransmitters via a series of specific ligands.
   C. PET resolution allows good visualization of small areas of cerebral activity.
   D. The radiation exposure in PET with FDG is minimal so that a subject can be studied several times a year if needed.
   E. PET with ^{15}O water has a long half-life, limiting the number of tasks participants can perform during scans.

9.3   Regarding SPECT, which of the following is true?

   A. SPECT has spatial resolution superior to that of PET.
   B. The radioligand [^{99m}Tc]hexamethylpropylene amine oxime (HMPAO) accumulates in endothelial cell membranes, but its activity remains constant for only 6 hours.
   C. Participants typically must receive radioligand injections in or near the scanning suite.
   D. SPECT is useful in diagnosis of dementia because it images neurodegeneration directly rather than inferring neural degeneration by decreased perfusion.
   E. Early SPECT studies using the cerebellum as a "control" region for cognitive processes must now be reinterpreted in light of the greater appreciation of the cognitive contribution of cerebellar function.

9.4 Regarding fMRI and MRS, which of the following is true?

    A. The mechanism of relative oxygen excess versus metabolic demands at the heart of fMRI has been well-defined.

    B. Oxygenated hemoglobin is more paramagnetic than deoxygenated and thus "looks brighter" on T_2-weighted pulse sequences.

    C. The clinical availability of fMRI is limited by its not being available in a conventional MRI scanner.

    D. MRS has similar spatial resolution to fMRI.

    E. MRS has been used to elucidate brain loss in neurodegenerative conditions via use of *N*-acetyl aspartate (NAA).

9.5 Functional neuroimaging has been used to assess findings in mood disorders. Which of the following is *not* true?

    A. Based on many functional neuroimaging studies of mood disorder patients, a region including the medial prefrontal cortex, perigenual cortex, posterior cingulate cortex, amygdala, and extended amygdala is typically affected.

    B. The medial prefrontal cortex, perigenual cortex, posterior cingulate cortex, amygdala, and extended amygdala circuit is also often implicated in anxiety disorders.

    C. Unipolar depressed patients with pseudodementia have been shown to have decreased blood flow to the left medial prefrontal cortex and increased flow to the cerebellum.

    D. Depressed patients were shown to have increases in metabolism of the prefrontal and anterior cingulate cortices following treatment.

    E. In studies of serotonin type 2 (5-HT$_2$) receptor, depressed patients had lower specific binding on PET; this specific binding increased with antidepressant treatment.

9.6 The functional neuroimaging of schizophrenia is more developed than for most other neuropsychiatric illnesses. Which of the following is *not* true?

    A. There is a graded response between dopamine type 2 (D$_2$) receptor occupancy (as evidenced by PET) and clinical findings, in which clinical response, prolactinemia, and extrapyramidal side effects were found at increasing levels of receptor occupancy by a typical antipsychotic medication.

    B. A SPECT study of olanzapine, low versus high doses, found a dose-dependent degree of D$_2$ receptor occupancy but no significant differences in clinical measures.

    C. Cerebellar dysfunction in schizophrenia has been demonstrated by an fMRI study showing decreased cerebellar blood flow in schizophrenic patients.

    D. Schizophrenic patients with hallucinations and delusions have been shown to have increased metabolism in the left temporal, inferior parietal, and occipital temporal regions.

    E. Schizophrenic patients with increased levels of cognitive and behavioral disorganization have been shown to have increased blood flow in the anterior cingulate cortex and contiguous medial prefrontal cortex, left superior temporal lobe, and thalamus.

C H A P T E R   1 0

Epidemiologic and Genetic Aspects of Neuropsychiatric Disorders

Select the single best response for each question.

10.1   Relative risk refers to the ratio of disease frequency in two different populations. The following five neuropsychiatric illnesses, all associated with cognitive impairment, have been found to have different relative risks when comparing morbid risk in first-degree relatives of affected patients to the rate of the illness in the general population. Which of these five illnesses has the lowest relative risk?

A.   Schizophrenia.
B.   Alzheimer's disease.
C.   Parkinson's disease.
D.   Huntington's disease.
E.   Pick's disease.

10.2   Which of the following types of study would be used by an investigator interested in identifying which chromosome is the site of a particular abnormal gene?

A.   Molecular approaches.
B.   Linkage analysis.
C.   High-risk studies.
D.   Segregation analysis.
E.   Pedigree analysis.

10.3   Regarding the genetic and epidemiological analysis of "complex disorders," all of the following are true *except*

A.   Many neuropsychiatric disorders feature a complex pattern of inheritance.
B.   The disorders exhibit incomplete penetrance, in which environmental factors may affect the degree to which a genetic disorder is phenotypically expressed.
C.   The disorders exhibit variable expressivity, in which a single form of the disorder may have different phenotypic expressions.
D.   Nonallelic heterogeneity refers to several genetic forms of a disorder following disruptions of a single gene.
E.   Anticipation refers to the decreased age at onset and increased severity of clinical disease of a single illness over successive generations.

10.4   Huntington's disease is a well-delineated genetic neuropsychiatric illness. Which of the following is true?

   A. The inheritance pattern is autosomal dominant with incomplete penetrance.
   B. Juvenile-onset Huntington's disease or the "Westphal variant" features akinesia and rigidity instead of chorea and has a more benign course.
   C. Common psychiatric symptoms include personality changes, dementia, psychosis, and depression; psychiatric symptoms may precede the onset of motor symptoms.
   D. Anticipation, in which subsequent generations have an earlier onset of illness, is more likely with maternal, rather than paternal, inheritance.
   E. Expanded CAG trinucleotide repeats on chromosome 4 are correlated with risk for disease and reliably predict age at onset of clinical symptoms in a given patient.

10.5   Parkinson's disease is another neuropsychiatric syndrome with significant epidemiologic and genetic considerations. Which of the following is true?

   A. Parkinson's disease features loss of pigmented neurons in the zona reticularis of the substantia nigra.
   B. Psychosis in Parkinson's disease is unrelated to advanced age or degree of cognitive decline.
   C. Worldwide studies consistently find that Caucasians have a greater risk for Parkinson's disease than people of African descent.
   D. Lewy bodies and Lewy neurites are pathological findings only in familial forms of Parkinson's disease.
   E. The α-synuclein gene on chromosome 4 has been linked to Lewy body production in early-onset Parkinson's disease.

10.6   Wilson's disease is a disorder of copper metabolism with dramatic neuropsychiatric symptoms. Which of the following is true?

   A. Wilson's disease features the failure of a single pathway in copper metabolism.
   B. Toxic amounts of copper accumulate in the liver and brain simultaneously.
   C. Other than the brain and liver, tissues affected by copper deposition include the kidney and iris.
   D. Siblings of affected patients, whose psychiatric symptoms include personality changes, depression, dementia, and psychosis, have a 25% risk of this disorder.
   E. The inheritance pattern is autosomal dominant with incomplete penetrance, and preclinical screening tests can aid in prophylactic treatment.

10.7   Which of the following is true regarding Alzheimer's disease?

   A. Cognitive impairment in Alzheimer's disease is more correlated with the presence of amyloid plaques, rather than tau-containing neurofibrillary tangles.
   B. Cerebrospinal fluid (CSF) analysis in Alzheimer's disease includes high β-amyloid protein and tau protein levels.
   C. Some epidemiological studies suggest both a protective effect of more education and an increased risk with lower levels of educational attainment.
   D. The apolipoprotein-E (APOE) gene represents the "susceptibility gene" for Alzheimer's disease, and its effects are similar on all ages and populations studied.
   E. In familial Alzheimer's disease, APOE ε4 homozygosity increases risk for illness but does not change age at onset.

10.8 Genetic linkage studies of bipolar disorder have identified several chromosomes with links to different variants of bipolar disorder. Which chromosome has been found in studies of the Old-Order Amish pedigree for bipolar disorder?

A. Chromosome 18.
B. Chromosome 21.
C. X chromosome.
D. Chromosome 11.
E. Chromosome 4.

10.9 Regarding genetic and epidemiological aspects of obsessive-compulsive disorder (OCD), which of the following is true?

A. There is a 15% excess of males as opposed to females.
B. Females have a significantly younger age at onset.
C. Affected females with early-onset illness have a higher incidence of birth complications than males.
D. Early onset predicts a higher incidence of Tourette's syndrome and other tic disorders in relatives.
E. Linkage analysis and genetic mode of inheritance for OCD are clearly established.

10.10 Schizophrenia has also been subjected to numerous genetic linkage studies. Which chromosome has been established as implicated in the failure of the sensory gating phenomenon in schizophrenia, based on the P50 auditory-evoked potential?

A. Chromosome 15.
B. Chromosome 13.
C. Chromosome 8.
D. Chromosome 22.
E. Chromosome 6.

C H A P T E R   1 1

Neuropsychiatric Aspects of Pain Management

Select the single best response for each question.

11.1   Which of the following is true regarding cognitive and emotional factors in pain?

   A.   Patients report more pain during the workweek than on weekends (because novelty enhances pain perception).
   B.   Reduced pain perception during hypnosis involves inhibition of the anterior cingulate gyrus.
   C.   Whereas pain patients score higher on measures of depression, anxiety is not notably increased in pain states.
   D.   Severe pain in oncology patients is strongly associated with symptoms of major depression.
   E.   In the Dworkin et al. (1990) study, even a single pain complaint was associated with a substantially increased risk for major depression.

11.2   Regarding the transduction of signals at peripheral sensory receptors, which of the following is true?

   A.   Mechanothermal receptors are the most common nociceptors.
   B.   Prostaglandins are known to directly excite pain fibers.
   C.   Polymodal C fiber receptors are likely responsible for transmission of "first pain" signals.
   D.   Cardiac muscle afferents can be stimulated by prostaglandins, histamine, and bradykinin.
   E.   Secondary hyperalgesia is primarily due to the actions of histamine, as serotonin does not affect peripheral nociceptors.

11.3   Regarding the spinal cord terminals of primary afferents and their projections, which of the following is true?

   A.   All somatic primary afferent cell bodies are in the dorsal root ganglia, adjacent to the spinal cord.
   B.   All primary afferent fibers terminate ipsilaterally in the dorsal gray matter.
   C.   Cells of lamina I are called marginal cells and are responsive to mechanical stimuli.
   D.   Lamina II is the nucleus proprius and is responsible for noxious stimuli, light touch, and pressure sense.
   E.   The spinothalamic tracts are composed of over 90% "crossed" fibers from laminae I, IV, V, VII, and VIII from the contralateral dorsal horn.

11.4   There are several opioid receptors with differential properties. Which of the following is *not* true regarding the μ opioid receptor?

    A. Agonists to the μ receptor induce pain relief.
    B. Agonists to the μ receptor decrease level of consciousness and may cause sedation.
    C. Agonists to the μ receptor may induce respiratory depression.
    D. Euphoric affect may follow μ receptor agonism.
    E. Pentazocine is a prototypical agonist of the μ receptor.

11.5   Regarding the use of antidepressants and other medications as pain adjuncts, which of the following is true?

    A. Among tricyclic antidepressants (TCAs), secondary amines are more effective at serotonin reuptake blockade, whereas tertiary amines are superior at norepinephrine reuptake blockade.
    B. Pain relief from antidepressants requires several weeks of dosing, as is true for relief of depression.
    C. Secondary amine antidepressants include nortriptyline, amitriptyline, and imipramine.
    D. Anticonvulsant drugs are likely to act by blocking voltage-dependent sodium channels in neurons and thus are indicated for neuropathic pain.
    E. Because of their generally more favorable side effect profile when compared with TCAs, selective serotonin reuptake inhibitors (SSRIs) now have a clearly established role in pain management.

11.6   Regarding the use of hypnosis in pain management, all of the following are true *except*

    A. Hypnosis works through two related mechanisms: peripheral muscle relaxation, and central perceptual alteration and cognitive distraction.
    B. Patients may be instructed to imagine that a painful body part is "numb."
    C. Patients may be told to imagine that painful tissue is "warm" or "cold" by using imagery.
    D. Research studies have demonstrated that hypnosis can result in a decreased need for pharmacological pain relief.
    E. Patients must be considered "highly hypnotizable" to have clinical relief from hypnosis for pain control.

11.7   The thalamus functions as a key "relay" center for the transmission of pain sensations. Which of the following is true?

    A. In the thalamus, spinothalamic neurons terminate primarily on the ventroposterolateral and submedius nuclei.
    B. The ventroposterolateral nucleus subserves the qualitative aspects of sensation.
    C. The centromedian nucleus is responsible for localization of impulses in space.
    D. Nucleus submedius functions are not clearly defined at this time.
    E. Projections from the ventroposterolateral nucleus to parietal lobe areas 1, 2, and 3 are central to the emotional aspects of pain sensation.

CHAPTER 12

Neuropsychiatric Aspects of Primary Headache Disorders

Select the single best response for each question.

12.1 Classification of headache according to the International Headache Society is important for clinical diagnosis and management. Which of the following symptoms would lead the clinician to rule out episodic tension-type headache?

    A. Nausea and vomiting.
    B. Pressing/tightening quality to the pain.
    C. Mild-moderate pain intensity; activities not prohibited by headache.
    D. Bilateral.
    E. Unaffected by routine physical activities.

12.2 Psychiatric comorbidity may be an important clinical consideration in the management of headache in patients. Which of the following is *not* true?

    A. A higher lifetime prevalence of major depression is seen in severe nonmigraine headache patients compared with headache-free patients.
    B. Depression is extremely common in patients with chronic migraine.
    C. Headache is a common physical complaint in depressed patients.
    D. Improvement in headache has not been shown to alter the patient's Minnesota Multiphasic Personality Inventory (MMPI) scores.
    E. Psychiatric comorbidity is associated with headache intractability.

12.3 The phenomenon of aura is an important consideration in many migraine patients. Which of the following is true regarding migraine aura?

    A. Over 50% of migraine patients experience auras.
    B. Aura is invariably followed by a headache.
    C. Visual auras may consist of "positive" symptoms (e.g., flashes of light) and "negative" symptoms (e.g., scotomata or blind spots).
    D. The fortification spectrum is an arc of scintillating lights that generally begins peripherally and then migrates centrally.
    E. Auras of paresthesias are most commonly experienced over the hemiface and in the contralateral upper extremity.

12.4 Basilar migraine may present an ambiguous clinical picture. Which of the following statements is true?

    A. Basilar migraine is seen only in persons younger than 30 years.
    B. Basilar migraine is more common in males than in females.
    C. Visual symptoms are characteristically bilateral at the onset of the aura.
    D. Unlike classic migraine, many of the symptoms are bilateral.
    E. Changes in cognitive status are unusual.

12.5 Regarding epidemiology and comorbidity of migraine, which of the following is true?

    A. Migraine and major depression are each associated with an increased prevalence of the other.
    B. The prevalence of migraine is greater for females than males throughout adult life, and this difference is greatest between ages 20 and 30 years.
    C. Migraine is more common with higher intelligence.
    D. Migraine increases the risk for epilepsy but not for stroke.
    E. Personality instruments have consistently shown that increased neuroticism predicts the presence of migraine in subjects of both sexes; these studies have not been contaminated by other psychiatric pathology and were all well-controlled.

12.6 Preventative treatment is often indicated for the migraine patient. Which of the following would *not* be considered a primary preventative treatment for migraine?

    A. β-Adrenergic blockers.
    B. Opioids.
    C. Antidepressants.
    D. Calcium-channel blockers.
    E. Anticonvulsants.

12.7 Cluster headache is a relatively rare but profoundly disabling condition. Which of the following is *not* a physical finding in cluster headache?

    A. Severe unilateral orbital, supraorbital, and temporal pain.
    B. Conjunctival injection.
    C. Lacrimation.
    D. Mydriasis.
    E. Ptosis.

12.8 Acute treatments for cluster headache include all of the following *except*

    A. Oxygen.
    B. Antipsychotics.
    C. Sumatriptan.
    D. Dihydroergotamine.
    E. Lidocaine.

C H A P T E R   1 3

Neuropsychiatric Aspects of Disorders of Attention

Select the single best response for each question.

13.1 *Executive control* involves the operation of several neurobehavioral systems. When a subject is able to efficiently shift from one response alternative to another to meet environmental demands, this phenomenon is called

   A. Intention.
   B. Selection.
   C. Initiation.
   D. Inhibition.
   E. Switching.

13.2 The neuroanatomical basis for attention involves several specific structures. Which of the following is *not* considered a key structure in attention?

   A. Reticular activating system (RAS).
   B. Thalamus and striatum.
   C. Dominant posterior parietal cortex.
   D. Prefrontal cortex.
   E. Limbic system.

13.3 The dorsolateral prefrontal cortex circuit is important in maintaining response flexibility and "working memory." Lesions of this system may result in all of the following *except*

   A. Perseveration.
   B. Distractibility.
   C. Cognitive slowing.
   D. Cognitive disorganization.
   E. Lability of affect.

13.4 The clinical assessment of attention may be assisted by the use of neuropsychological test instruments. Which of the following is a test of response selection and control or executive control?

   A. Wisconsin Card Sorting Test.
   B. Weschler Adult Intelligence Scale—Revised (WAIS-R): picture completion.
   C. Stroop Test.
   D. Paced Auditory Serial Addition Task.
   E. Continuous Performance Test.

13.5   The assessment and classification of the level of consciousness are important to accomplish in an orderly and standardized fashion. If the patient exhibits spontaneous eye opening, eye opening in response to pain, roving eye movements, and/or blink in response to threat, but no awareness or meaningful responsiveness, this would be considered to be

A. Locked-in syndrome.
B. Akinetic mutism.
C. Persistent vegetative state.
D. Stupor.
E. Confusional state.

13.6   Hemineglect can be formulated as a unilateral attentional disorder. All of the following are true of the hemineglect syndrome *except*

A. Patients fail to draw the left half of a drawing.
B. Patients have measurable (though not complete) hemianopia on formal visual field testing.
C. Patients may have hemisomatosensory neglect.
D. Patients may deny "ownership" of the extremities in the neglected hemispace.
E. Neglect affecting several sensory modalities supports the model of neglect as an attentional, rather than a perceptual, disorder.

13.7   Which of the following is true regarding attentional deficits and major depression?

A. Depressed patients rarely complain of difficulty in focus and concentration.
B. Focused attention and sustained attention are less likely to be reduced in depression than sensory selective attention.
C. Attentional performance in depression remains static over time.
D. Manic patients make errors typified by poor inhibition and errors of "commission," whereas depressed patients have low arousal and make errors of "omission."
E. Depression rarely needs to be ruled out when evaluating other attentional disorders.

13.8   Which is true regarding attention-deficit/hyperactivity disorder (ADHD)?

A. Between 30% and 50% of child ADHD patients continue with disabling symptoms in adulthood.
B. There may be wide cultural variance in the diagnosis of ADHD; for example, ADHD is diagnosed 10 times more often in North America than in Great Britain.
C. Most ADHD patients have cognitive impairment on formal assessment.
D. Poor performance on WAIS-R Digit Span, Arithmetic, and Digit Symbol subtests is pathognomonic for ADHD.
E. Errors of both "omission" and "commission" are characteristic of ADHD subjects.

C H A P T E R   1 4

Neuropsychiatric Aspects of Delirium

Select the single best response for each question.

14.1   Patients with delirium can present with a multiplicity of clinical appearances. Regarding the signs and symptoms of delirium, which of the following is true?

A. The majority of delirium patients manifest the "hyperactive" or agitated type.

B. The distinction between delirium and Lewy body dementia is often clear because of the rare presence of prominent psychotic symptoms in Lewy body dementia.

C. Delirium is more common in dementia due to Pick's disease and Lewy body dementia than in dementia due to Alzheimer's disease and vascular dementia.

D. Delirium in a patient with dementia has a substantially different presentation than delirium in a patient without dementia.

E. Diffuse electroencephalographic slowing is more than twice as common in delirium as in dementia and can thus assist the physician in differential diagnosis.

14.2   Regarding the epidemiology and morbidity/mortality of delirium, all of the following are true *except*

A. Studies of the epidemiology of delirium have shown a 10-fold difference in incidence and prevalence rates in hospitalized patients.

B. More than 10% of elderly patients may be expected to be delirious on hospital admission, and nearly 50% are delirious at some point during hospitalization.

C. Hyperactive delirium has been consistently found to have a higher mortality rate than hypoactive or mixed types.

D. Excess mortality in delirium patients may be somewhat attributable to excessive age, dementia, or other systemic morbidity compared with nondelirious patients.

E. Increased rates on institutionalization and decreased independent community living have been frequently found following episodes of delirium.

14.3   The concept of delirium risk factors and precipitant events has important consequences for clinical management. Which of the following is true?

A. Medication exposure is a factor in less than 20% of cases of delirium.

B. Standardized protocols to assess cognition, sleep, sensory deprivation, and hydration status have been shown to reduce the number, but not duration, of delirium episodes.

C. Postoperative delirium is most common on the first postoperative day.

D. Low albumin level may predispose a patient to delirium, in part by increasing the bioavailability of medications.

E. Increased blood-brain barrier permeability predisposes to delirium, but this is of clinical importance only with central nervous system surgery, illness, or injury.

14.4 Anticholinergic activity (expressed in terms of atropine equivalents) is an important property in a medication's propensity to induce delirium. Among the following common medications, which one has the highest level of anticholinergic activity?

A. Prednisolone.
B. Cimetidine.
C. Ranitidine.
D. Theophylline.
E. Furosemide.

14.5 Formal cognitive assessment is crucial in the evaluation of delirium. Which of the following is true?

A. The Mini-Mental State Exam (MMSE) is useful to establish the presence of a cognitive disorder and reliably distinguishes delirium from dementia.
B. A weakness of the MMSE is its lack of items that directly assess frontal lobe and nondominant hemisphere functions.
C. The clock drawing test screens for cognitive disorders and distinguishes delirium from dementia.
D. The Confusion Assessment Method requires administration by a psychiatrist.
E. The Delirium Rating Scale—Revised–98 reliably distinguishes delirium from dementia and functions well with repeated measures.

14.6 The electroencephalogram (EEG) may be a helpful adjunctive test for delirium. The most characteristic delirium pattern on EEG is diffuse slowing. Which EEG pattern is seen with delirium tremens from alcohol withdrawal?

A. Low-voltage fast activity.
B. Diffuse slowing.
C. Spikes/polyspikes, frontocentral.
D. Left/bilateral slowing or delta bursts.
E. Epileptiform activity, frontotemporal or generalized.

14.7 Delirium symptoms have been found to vary across different studies. In attempts to unify the clinical diagnosis of delirium, a Trzepacz (1999) study grouped symptoms into "core" and "associated" or "noncore" symptoms. Which of the following is considered an associated or noncore symptom?

A. Attentional deficits.
B. Memory impairment.
C. Perceptual disturbances.
D. Thought process abnormality.
E. Motoric alterations.

14.8 Regarding psychopharmacological management of delirium, which of the following is true?

A. Physostigmine is an attractive medication to reverse anticholinergic delirium and has a safe side-effect profile.
B. Haloperidol must be used with caution in hemodynamically unstable patients on pressor support because it can reverse dopamine-induced increases in renal blood flow.
C. Because of QT_c prolongation risk with haloperidol, it should not be used in patients with QT_c greater than 400 msec.
D. As an alternative to haloperidol, intravenous droperidol can be used, although it can induce hypotension due to α-adrenergic agonism.
E. Among atypical antipsychotics, clozapine is contraindicated in delirium because of its anticholinergic effects.

CHAPTER 15

Neuropsychiatric Aspects of Aphasia and Related Disorders

Select the single best response for each question.

15.1   The clinical aphasias are classified according to functional deficits according to the model of Wernicke-Geschwind. Which of the following is true?

    A. Writing comprehension is preserved in most aphasia syndromes.

    B. Anomic aphasia can be usually differentiated from Wernicke's aphasia in that only the former has impaired naming of common objects.

    C. Conduction and Wernicke's aphasia both feature fluent speech with notable paraphasic speech errors.

    D. Transcortical motor aphasia and transcortical sensory aphasia can be reliably differentiated by the presence of normal speech fluency in the former.

    E. Global aphasia, despite several functional speech defects, generally features preserved fluency.

15.2   For the examination of language function in the Wernicke-Geschwind model, which of the following is considered a major language area?

    A. Word-list generation.

    B. Repetition.

    C. Automatic speech.

    D. Prosody.

    E. Speech mechanics.

15.3   Broca's and Wernicke's aphasias are two of the aphasia syndromes best known to most psychiatrists. Which of the following is true?

    A. Despite being caused by a left-sided cortical lesion, apraxia of the left upper extremity and buccal-lingual apraxia are common.

    B. Prognosis for functional recovery may depend on the "depth" of the central nervous system lesion; cortical lesions are generally permanent, whereas internal capsule lesions tend to produce reversible aphasia.

    C. Patients with Wernicke's aphasia generally experience a loss of normal speech prosody.

    D. Because of the posterior superior temporal lobe of the left cortex location of the lesion in Wernicke's aphasia, a left inferior quadrantanopsia may be seen.

    E. In the poststroke patient, the clinician may have to differentiate Wernicke's aphasia from delirium. The delirium patient will often exhibit speed with empty content, whereas the Wernicke's aphasia patient will be incoherent.

15.4   The syndromes of conduction aphasia and global aphasia may be encountered less often than Broca's and Wernicke's aphasias. Which of the following is true?

    A. In conduction aphasia, repetition and naming are affected similarly.
    B. In conduction aphasia, reading comprehension is invariably abnormal.
    C. In conduction aphasia, when present, apraxia is limited to the right upper extremity.
    D. Global aphasia refers to deficits in all language modalities and is often accompanied by a right hemiplegia, right hemisensory deficit, and right homonymous hemianopsia.
    E. Because of the magnitude of deficits, global aphasia can only follow an infarction in the distribution of the middle cerebral artery from a single devastating stroke.

15.5   Which of the following is true regarding other aphasia syndromes and the analogous condition of aprosodia?

    A. Transcortical motor aphasia is clinically similar to Broca's aphasia except that the patient retains the ability to repeat accurately.
    B. Transcortical sensory aphasia features paraphasic errors but not echolalia.
    C. Anomic aphasia is a specific syndrome with defined neuroanatomical location and is unrelated to other aphasia syndromes.
    D. Patients with anomic aphasias rarely experience alexia and agraphia in addition to anomia.
    E. The aprosodia patient's emotionless response more resembles a psychotic disorder than a mood disorder.

15.6   The psychiatric comorbidity of aphasia syndromes may have important clinical consequences. Which of the following is true?

    A. The frustration of the Broca's aphasia patient in efforts at communication may lead to agitated gestures and expletives.
    B. Depression is equally common in anterior- and posterior-hemisphere lesions that lead to aphasia.
    C. Because of the frustration over communication failure and depression, suicide risk is particularly high in Broca's aphasia.
    D. Posterior aphasia behavioral syndrome features mood disturbance but rarely psychosis.
    E. Patients with posterior aphasia, despite other comprehension problems, usually can recognize their own recorded speech.

CHAPTER 16

Neuropsychiatric Aspects of Aggression and Impulse Control Disorders

Select the single best response for each question.

16.1 Regarding the epidemiology of violent behavior in the United States, which of the following is true?

A. Homicide is the leading cause of death of people ages 15–24 years.
B. Women are equally likely as men to die by homicide.
C. In cases of domestic violence, men are more likely to attack their domestic partner than are women.
D. In 50% of homicides, both perpetrator and victim are of the same race.
E. Nations with strict gun control laws have lower homicide rates than does the United States.

16.2 Clinical assessment instruments may assist the clinician in evaluation and management of the violent patient. Which of the following is true?

A. Despite the development of more specific instruments, the Rorschach and Thematic Apperception tests remain definitive tests for evaluating aggressive behavior.
B. The Buss-Durkee Hostility Inventory requires clinician administration.
C. The Hostility and Direction of Hostility Questionnaire (HDHQ) is derived from components of the broader Millon Clinical Multiaxial Inventory.
D. The Brown-Goodwin Assessment (BGA) is clinician administered and includes clinical interview and review of available records.
E. The BGA contains 11 assessments, all of which address physical aggression against others.

16.3 Research has addressed the putative roles of various central nervous system structures in aggressive behavior. Which of the following statements is true?

A. Adults who have experienced physical abuse are much more likely to exhibit violent behavior as adults, a behavior that is directly related to the effects of head injury.
B. Destruction of the ventromedial nucleus of the hypothalamus in animal models leads to passive behavior.
C. Hamsters exhibit aggressive behavior after the administration of arginine vasopressin in the hypothalamus; this effect is blunted by the coadministration of a 5-hydroxytryptamine (serotonin) type 1B ($5-HT_{1B}$) receptor agonist.
D. In animal models, stimulation of the amygdala has a variable effect on aggression, depending on the animal's preexisting temperament.
E. Patients with temporal lobe epilepsy are more likely to demonstrate aggressive behavior in the ictal or immediate postictal period than in the interictal period.

16.4 The prefrontal cortex has garnered a great deal of attention in the study of aggression. Which of the following is true?

    A. As with temporal lobe epilepsy patients who behave violently, patients with frontal lobe injury and violent behavior typically show remorse for their violent acts after the fact.

    B. Orbital lesions of the prefrontal cortex often result in impaired long-term planning and increased apathy.

    C. Dorsal prefrontal lesions are associated with increased affective responses to stimuli encountered in the environment.

    D. According to Soloff et al. (2000), patients with narcissistic personality disorder had a diminished response to serotonergic stimulation in prefrontal areas subserving behavioral regulation.

    E. According to Raine et al. (1998), subjects who committed impulsive murders had impaired prefrontal cortex function when compared with predatory (nonimpulsive) murderers.

16.5 Much study of the neurochemistry of aggressive behavior has focused on the effects of serotonin. Which of the following is true?

    A. Suicidal depressed patients have been found to have lower cerebrospinal fluid (CSF) 5-hydroxyindoleacetic acid (5-HIAA; a serotonin metabolite) levels than depressed patients without suicidality.

    B. Among patients with Axis I disorders, CSF 5-HIAA levels are decreased in aggressive patients only if they also exhibit suicidal behavior.

    C. The Linnoila et al. (1983) study cited demonstrated that decreased CSF 5-HIAA was decreased in all violent behavior, irrespective of premeditation.

    D. Decreased brainstem levels in suicide victims have been reported in several studies, but this finding has been inconsistent across different studies.

    E. Increased platelet transporter sites for serotonin, reflecting serotonin deficiency, are commonly seen in aggressive psychiatric patients.

16.6 Which of the following is true regarding the neuropsychological and neuropsychiatric aspects of violent behavior and other clinical findings?

    A. There is broad support for the finding that borderline personality disorder with violent behavior is solely a consequence of cognitive impairment.

    B. Selective serotonin reuptake inhibitors (SSRIs) have been shown to decrease violent behavior but have not been shown to decrease nonviolent impulsive behavior (e.g., problematic gambling).

    C. Paroxetine is the most thoroughly studied SSRI for impulsive behavior in borderline personality disorder.

    D. High-dose fluoxetine in borderline personality disorder has been associated with decreased self-injurious behavior.

    E. Tricyclic antidepressants have been consistently shown to be effective for aggression and impulsivity in borderline personality disorder, similar to their effects on depression.

CHAPTER 17

Neuropsychiatric Aspects of Memory and Amnesia

Select the single best response for each question.

17.1 Regarding conceptual classification of memory systems, which of the following memory functions is considered a component of working memory?

    A. Central executive or "scratch pad."
    B. Semantic.
    C. Episodic.
    D. Procedural.
    E. Conditioning.

17.2 The acquisition of memory about the environment that is not cued to specific personal experiences and cannot be fixed as having been acquired at a discrete point in time is referred to as which type of memory?

    A. Episodic.
    B. Semantic.
    C. Procedural.
    D. Priming.
    E. Conditioning.

17.3 Which of the following is true regarding specific memory functions?

    A. Procedural memory refers to the acquisition of motor, but not cognitive, skills.
    B. Procedural memory requires intact hippocampal function.
    C. Physiological and environmental manipulations, such as cooling or central nervous system anoxia, disrupt short-term and long-term memory to an equal degree.
    D. Electroconvulsive therapy (ECT)–induced amnesia's general transient nature supports the concept that memory retrieval, rather than storage, is affected by ECT.
    E. Animal models with disruption in messenger ribonucleic acid (mRNA) synthesis decrease both short-term and long-term memory.

17.4 Although they are not invariably present in all patients with amnestic disorders, the four clinical characteristics of amnestic disorders include all of the following clinical symptoms *except*

    A. Anterograde amnesia.
    B. Retrograde amnesia.
    C. Behavioral disinhibition or personality change.
    D. Confabulation.
    E. Relatively preserved intellectual function in other domains.

17.5   Which is true regarding Wernicke-Korsakoff syndrome?

   A. The syndrome is caused by lesions of the temporal lobes, whereas the diencephalon is spared.
   B. The acute phase, Wernicke's encephalopathy, classically features acute mental status changes, gait disturbances, oculomotor disturbances, and mononeuropathy.
   C. The chronic phase, Korsakoff's psychosis, requires active hallucinations and/or delusions for diagnosis.
   D. Dense anterograde amnesia and gradient retrograde amnesia are seen in the Korsakoff's stage of the illness.
   E. Formal neuropsychological assessment generally reveals intact visuoperceptual and spatial organization functions, despite amnesia.

17.6   Depressed patients may present with memory complaints and/or findings of amnesia on clinical examination. Which of the following is true?

   A. Depressed patients with attention and concentration deficits may have impaired working memory as evidenced by the digit-span test.
   B. Despite complaints of memory dysfunction, depressed patients do not show defects in recall or recognition on formal testing.
   C. Depressed patients will generally complain of similar degrees of memory dysfunction on both "effortful" and "automatic" cognitive tasks.
   D. Depressed patients have greater difficulty with nondeclarative memory than with declarative memory.
   E. Depressed patients have greater access to pleasant than to unpleasant memories.

17.7   Regarding the syndrome of transient global amnesia (TGA), which of the following is true?

   A. Patients are usually elderly.
   B. The anterograde component of amnesia resolves before the retrograde component.
   C. During the amnestic period, disorientation (even to personal identity) is typical.
   D. Functional neuroimaging of TGA patients has shown transient decreased metabolic and functional activity in mesial temporal lobe structures.
   E. Cognitive functions other than memory are typically abnormal during an attack of TGA.

17.8   Amnesia following ECT treatments is a troubling side effect of this intervention. Which of the following is true?

   A. Differences in cognitive effects between bilateral and unilateral ECT treatments tend to be persistent, even well after the end of the ECT course of treatment.
   B. ECT typically degrades both declarative and procedural memory.
   C. There is a predictable, dose-response relationship between efficacy of ECT for mood disorders and the likelihood of postprocedural amnesia.
   D. Recent research suggests that patients most prone to post-ECT persistent retrograde amnesia are more likely to have had preexisting cognitive impairment.
   E. In post-ECT retrograde amnesia, memory for public events is less than for personal events.

C H A P T E R   1 8

Neuropsychiatric Aspects of Traumatic Brain Injury

Select the single best response for each question.

18.1 The pathophysiology of traumatic brain injury (TBI) has been examined from the perspectives of cellular metabolism and specific neuroanatomic vulnerability. Which of the following statements is true?

A. In TBI, damaged neurons have an acute metabolic need for increased blood flow, but the postinjury increase in blood flow is inadequate to meet these needs.

B. Secondary neurotoxicity includes calcium efflux, phospholipase activation, excitotoxin release, and lipid peroxidation.

C. One of the excitotoxic neurotransmitters in secondary neurotoxicity, glutamate, is increased in the cerebrospinal fluid (CSF) of TBI patients.

D. Hippocampal vulnerability to the effects of TBI is due to its predilection for damage by hypoxia and elevated intracranial pressure.

E. Functional alterations in hippocampal lesions correlate with decrements in memory and require cell death.

18.2 The Glasgow Coma Scale (GCS) is a useful tool for clinical classification of neuropsychiatric functioning. Which of the following is true of assessment of TBI with the GCS?

A. Scores on the GCS range from 0 to 15.

B. Mild TBI is indicated by a GCS of 13–15 with loss of consciousness from 5 to 20 minutes.

C. Severe TBI requires a GCS of 8 or less, with abnormal findings on all three components of the scale.

D. *Decerebrate* posturing is considered a higher level of motor response than *decorticate* posturing.

E. The GCS is useful for both initial and follow-up assessment of level of neurologic function.

18.3 Neuroimaging by various modalities is often important in the evaluation and management of TBI. Which of the following statements is *not* true?

A. Because the radiographic density of central nervous system (CNS) lesions may evolve, it is not uncommon for a computed tomography (CT) scan obtained 3 months after the head injury to reveal lesions initially unseen.

B. The frontal and temporal lobes are frequently the site of CNS lesions resulting in neuropsychiatric symptoms and are better visualized by magnetic resonance imaging (MRI) than CT.

C. MRI with morphometric analysis may demonstrate hippocampal atrophy and decreased thalamic volume in TBI.

D. MRI is preferred to CT for the imaging of contusions and subdural and epidural hematomas.

E. Single photon emission computed tomography (SPECT) should be used preferentially to CT and MRI where it is available.

18.4 Regarding various neuropsychiatric clinical features associated with TBI, which of the following is true?

A. Anosmia, as manifest by deficiency in olfactory naming and recognition, may correlate with frontal and/or temporal lobe injury but is not of prognostic importance.

B. Substance abuse is associated with greater morbidity, but not mortality, from TBI.

C. Similar to the epidemiology of Alzheimer's disease, presence of the apolipoprotein-E (APOE) ε4 allele is associated with poorer functional recovery in TBI.

D. Personality changes following TBI are significant in a minority of patients.

E. TBI with damage to the orbitofrontal cortex results in a condition similar to the "negative/deficit" state of schizophrenia, with cognitive slowness, apathy, and perseveration.

18.5 Mood disorders may follow TBI. Which of the following is true?

A. Patients with TBI do not differ significantly from noninjured patients with regard to their preinjury history of psychiatric illness.

B. The Beck Depression Inventory (BDI) is a reliable indicator of depression following TBI, even in the absence of formal psychiatric examination.

C. The increased suicide risk in TBI is primarily because of the incidence of major depression, with disinhibition from frontal lobe injury a minor factor.

D. The increased risk of depression after TBI has been shown to be approximately 25% at 1, 3, 6, and 12 months post-TBI.

E. The risk of depression after TBI is linearly related to duration of peri-injury loss of consciousness and duration of posttraumatic amnesia and is increased if there was skull fracture.

18.6 Mild TBI has been associated with a constellation of neuropsychiatric symptoms called postconcussion syndrome. Which of the following is true?

A. Whereas the mechanism of injury is primarily diffuse axonal injury, neither structural (e.g., CT, MRI) nor functional (e.g., electroencephalogram, SPECT) assessments reveal abnormalities in mild TBI.

B. Whereas many postconcussion patients may complain of cognitive symptoms, these can infrequently be detected on formal neuropsychological examination at 3-month follow-up.

C. The majority of mild TBI patients recover cognitive function and experience decreased symptoms by 6 months.

D. Compensation for injury and ongoing litigation adversely affect recovery from mild TBI.

E. In the case of concurrent postconcussion symptoms and posttraumatic stress disorder (PTSD), PTSD symptoms typically spontaneously reverse earlier.

18.7 Psychopharmacological therapy may be invaluable in the management of symptoms following TBI. Which of the following is true?

A. Because of increased blood-brain barrier permeability and greater CSF penetration of psychotropic agents, both the starting and final doses of medications in TBI should be less than those for a neurologically intact adult.

B. Because of the likelihood of persistent risk for depressed mood in TBI, antidepressants generally should be continued indefinitely.

C. Because of the risk of additional amnestic symptoms, even with shorter courses of electroconvulsive therapy (ECT), ECT is discouraged in TBI patients.

D. Antidepressants are indicated for "pathological emotions" in TBI patients, even in the absence of a full-spectrum mood disorder.

E. Because they have been shown to dramatically increase the risk of seizures in TBI patients, psychostimulants are to be used only with great caution and with concurrent anticonvulsant therapy.

18.8 Many medication classes are recommended for both acute and chronic management of persistently agitated/aggressive behavior in TBI. Which of the following medication classes is *not* recommended for the management of chronic agitation?

A. Benzodiazepines.

B. Atypical antipsychotics.

C. β-Blockers.

D. Buspirone.

E. Anticonvulsants.

CHAPTER 19

Neuropsychiatric Aspects of Seizure Disorders

Select the single best response for each question.

19.1   Which of the following is true regarding the International League Against Epilepsy (ILAE) classification scheme for seizure types?

   A. The anatomical locus for seizure syndromes (e.g., temporal lobe epilepsy) is preserved.
   B. The classification categorizes seizure syndromes, taking into account epidemiological variables such as age, sex, and concurrent illness.
   C. The main classification "branching" according to this scheme is partial versus focal seizures.
   D. Seizures that begin as partial seizures and then evolve to generalized tonic-clonic seizures are considered to then be "generalized."
   E. Absence seizures are considered focal because they do not have a notable motor component in most cases.

19.2   Which of the following is true regarding specific seizure syndromes?

   A. Complex partial seizures (CPSs) are experienced by a majority of seizure disorder patients.
   B. Absence seizures occur primarily in children and feature bilateral, synchronous electroencephalogram (EEG) spike waves between 6 and 7 Hz.
   C. When CPSs and absence seizures persist in status epilepticus, this represents a medical emergency, as is the case with tonic-clonic seizure status epilepticus.
   D. Temporal lobe epilepsy as a clinical syndrome is synonymous with CPSs.
   E. Temporal lobe seizures may be associated with 10–30 seconds of loss of consciousness accompanied by behavioral automatisms.

19.3   The clinical diagnosis of seizure disorder typically requires support from laboratory, neuroimaging, and EEG data. Which of the following is true regarding the findings in seizure disorder?

   A. The EEG is a definitive test, as over 90% of seizure disorder patients have abnormal EEGs, most often with "spike and wave" tracings.
   B. Increased serum prolactin, typically 3–4 times the patient's baseline level, is seen with equal frequency with generalized tonic-clonic seizures and partial complex seizures.
   C. Functional neuroimaging may be helpful, although single photon emission computed tomography (SPECT) is superior to positron emission tomography (PET) in the localization of interictal temporal lobe hypermetabolism.
   D. Clinical yield of EEG can be increased by placement of nasopharyngeal and sphenoidal electrodes, and both of these techniques equally increase the detection of seizure foci.
   E. A sleep EEG greatly increases the detection of focal abnormalities, such as a temporal lobe seizure focus.

19.4 Nonepileptic seizures or "pseudoseizures" may complicate the clinical management of a patient with an apparent seizure disorder. Which of the following is true of pseudoseizure patients?

  A. The patients commonly also experience dissociative disorders rather than somatoform disorders.
  B. The seizures are often related to sleep.
  C. Motor symptoms have a characteristic abrupt onset and sudden remission.
  D. Neurological reflexes are preserved.
  E. Minor injury is common, as patients attempt to persuade the examiner of the legitimacy of seizures.

19.5 The appearance of psychotic symptoms with seizure syndromes may render diagnosis and clinical management problematic. Which of the following is true regarding the differential diagnosis of psychotic symptoms in seizure disorders?

  A. Some seizure patients experience periodic perceptual changes, alterations in level of consciousness, and intact memory for seizure events.
  B. A chronic psychotic condition related to seizure disorder typically features complex hallucinations in several sensory modalities.
  C. Seizure-related psychotic symptoms are generally communicated as being ego-syntonic.
  D. Patients with atypical psychoses (i.e., psychotic conditions not clearly meeting criteria for schizophrenia) are more likely to have comorbid epilepsy than schizophrenic patients.
  E. Among the atypical antipsychotic agents, clozapine is no more likely to lower the seizure threshold than other atypical agents.

19.6 The differential diagnosis of seizure symptoms includes symptoms of various anxiety disorders. Which of the following is true?

  A. There is a strong epidemiological association between seizure disorder and panic disorder, based on the presence of overlapping symptoms.
  B. Dissociative symptoms are more characteristic of seizure disorders than of anxiety disorders, thus usually they can be used by the clinician to distinguish between the two illnesses.
  C. A positive family history is much more likely in seizure disorder than in panic disorder.
  D. Attacks of CPSs are usually shorter than panic attacks.
  E. Anxiety due to seizure disorder will typically respond to antidepressants.

19.7 Comorbid mood disorders may complicate management of seizure disorders. Which of the following is true?

  A. Patients with temporal lobe epilepsy have a modestly increased risk of suicidal behavior.
  B. Neurosurgery for refractory temporal lobe seizures has been associated with a decreased recurrence of comorbid depression.
  C. Seizures following the use of antidepressants is an idiosyncratic, rather than dose-related, phenomenon.
  D. Treatment of depression in seizure patients rarely improves seizure control per se.
  E. Selective serotonin reuptake inhibitors have been shown to be superior to other antidepressants for mood disorders in seizure patients and thus should be used preferentially.

C H A P T E R   2 0

Neuropsychiatric Aspects of Sleep and Sleep Disorders

Select the single best response for each question.

20.1 Which of the following is true regarding sleep stages and their electroencephalogram (EEG) correlates?

A. Sleep onset is determined when the alpha wave activity increases to greater than 50% of a given epoch (30 seconds of recording time).
B. Stage II sleep features sleep spindles and/or K complexes, with delta-wave activity representing less than 20% of an epoch.
C. Stage III sleep requires delta-wave activity for greater than 50% of an epoch.
D. Stages I–IV are called non–rapid eye movement (NREM) sleep, whereas slow-wave sleep refers to Stage IV and REM.
E. Young adults typically spend one-third of the night in REM sleep.

20.2 *Sleep architecture* refers to the progression of sleep through various stages during a sleep period. Which of the following is true?

A. Sleep onset in normal healthy subjects is into REM sleep.
B. NREM and REM sleep alternate approximately every 180 minutes.
C. Slow-wave sleep is predominant in the late part of a sleep period.
D. REM sleep is predominant in the early part of a sleep cycle.
E. Slow-wave sleep decreases with age and can even disappear with time.

20.3 Sleep complaints can be important features in many neuropsychiatric disorders. Which of the following is true?

A. Approximately 20% of patients with a main complaint of insomnia have a psychiatric illness.
B. Selective REM deprivation can be used to treat depression.
C. Antidepressant medications increase REM sleep and suppress NREM sleep.
D. Unlike other antidepressants, bupropion and trazodone suppress REM sleep.
E. Patients with schizophrenia have excess rebound REM sleep following REM sleep deprivation.

20.4 Periodic limb movement disorder (PLMD) is a troubling condition for many patients. Which of the following is true?

A. This condition was previously called nocturnal myoclonus.
B. The upper extremities are more commonly affected than the lower extremities.
C. Despite the limb movements, patients are not aroused out of sleep.
D. PLMD occurs as a disturbance of paralysis during REM.
E. Antidepressants are associated with decreased limb movements.

20.5 Regarding pharmacological treatment of insomnia and related complaints, which of the following is true?

    A. Because of its high abuse potential, clonazepam is rarely prescribed for PLMD.

    B. Tricyclic antidepressants (TCAs) have little effect on slow-wave sleep, whereas selective serotonin reuptake inhibitors (SSRIs) increase it.

    C. Monoamine oxidase inhibitors (MAOIs) suppress both slow-wave sleep and REM sleep.

    D. Benzodiazepines have a more dramatic effect on slow-wave sleep than on REM sleep.

    E. The major advantage of newer-generation hypnotic agents (e.g., zolpidem) is the absence of memory impairment associated with their use.

20.6 Which of the following is *not* a risk factor for the sleep apnea syndrome?

    A. Male sex.

    B. Middle age or older.

    C. Obesity.

    D. Micrognathia.

    E. Hyperthyroidism.

20.7 The parasomnias are a group of sleep behavior disorders that are conceptualized by overlapping of various sleep cycles. Which of the following is true?

    A. A patient with sleepwalking is generally easily awakened during an episode of sleepwalking.

    B. Patients with sleep terrors are usually troubled by vivid memories of the terror episode.

    C. Nightmares are more common in patients with schizotypal, schizoid, and borderline personality disorder.

    D. Bruxism is most common in stage III and stage IV sleep.

    E. REM sleep behavior can be distinguished from sleepwalking in that the REM sleep behavior patient is "aware" of the actual physical environment, whereas the sleepwalker is not.

CHAPTER 21

Neuropsychiatric Aspects of Cerebrovascular Disorders

Select the single best response for each question.

21.1 Cerebrovascular disease leading to neuropsychiatric illness may arise from a number of pathophysiological mechanisms. Which of the following is true?

   A. Atherosclerotic thrombosis is approximately twice as common as cerebral embolism as a cause of stroke.
   B. Transient ischemic attacks are equally common with thrombosis and embolism.
   C. Cardiac sources of cerebral emboli commonly include arrhythmias, congenital heart disease, prosthetic valves, and myocardial infarction.
   D. Lacunae affecting the small penetrating cerebral arteries commonly produce mixed motor and sensory strokes.
   E. Intracerebral hemorrhage is accompanied by a severe, throbbing headache in nearly 90% of cases.

21.2 Cerebrovascular disease is associated with a series of systemic disturbances referred to as *multiple vascular risk factors*. Which of the following is *not* considered a risk factor for atherosclerotic thrombosis?

   A. Alcoholism.
   B. Hyperlipidemia.
   C. Diabetes mellitus.
   D. Hypertension.
   E. Cigarette smoking.

21.3 Various neuropsychiatric syndromes have been described in association with cerebrovascular disease. Which of the following is true?

   A. Major depression is associated with left frontal lobe and basal ganglia lesions, with strongest hemispheric correlation of risk occurring 6 months after cerebrovascular accident (CVA).
   B. Minor depression, subsyndromal for major depression, is approximately three times more common than major depression after CVA.
   C. Unlike depressive disorders, poststroke anxiety disorders are more common with right-sided CVA.
   D. Poststroke apathy is more common as part of a poststroke depression (PSD) than as an isolated neuropsychiatric symptom.
   E. Pathological laughter and/or crying poststroke have a similar prevalence to major depression.

21.4   PSD is the most thoroughly studied post-CVA neuropsychiatric illness. Which of the following is true regarding the phenomenology and clinical presentation of PSD?

   A.   Because of symptom overlap with physical causes of specific symptoms attributable to PSD, DSM-IV criteria must be modified for the accurate diagnosis of PSD.
   B.   According to a study by Lipsey et al. (1986; quoted in Robinson 1998), PSD and functional major depression patients had nearly identical symptom profiles.
   C.   Poststroke catastrophic reaction and hyperemotionalism are integral to the diagnosis of PSD.
   D.   According to PSD epidemiological studies, PSD is more common in community settings than in hospital settings.
   E.   PSD persists beyond 1 year in the majority of cases.

21.5   Premorbid risk factors and comorbid physical and/or cognitive impairment may be important variables in the clinical management of PSD. Which of the following is true?

   A.   Cortical atrophy appears to be a greater risk factor for PSD than subcortical atrophy.
   B.   A family history of depression is more common in PSD patients with left-sided than right-sided CVA or nondepressed CVA patients.
   C.   Poor functional recovery leads to increased risk of PSD more than does PSD lead to poor functional recovery.
   D.   Patients with PSD are more likely than nondepressed CVA patients to exhibit post-CVA cognitive impairment; this relationship appears stronger for left-sided lesions.
   E.   PSD treatment studies have consistently shown improved cognition following successful antidepressant therapy.

21.6   Regarding randomized, placebo-controlled, double-blind treatment studies for PSD, which of the following is true?

   A.   Nortriptyline showed greater improvement than placebo for PSD without cognitive side effects requiring discontinuation of treatment in the active drug patients.
   B.   Trazodone was shown to improve Hamilton Rating Scale for Depression (Ham-D) scores in PSD more than did placebo.
   C.   The first SSRI with demonstrated efficacy for PSD was citalopram.
   D.   Fluoxetine was shown to be equally effective to nortriptyline for PSD.
   E.   Fluoxetine and nortriptyline were both associated with weight loss in PSD treatment.

21.7   Which of the following antidepressants have been shown to be effective in the treatment of pathologic emotions after stroke?

   A.   Nortriptyline and fluoxetine.
   B.   Fluoxetine and citalopram.
   C.   Sertraline and nortriptyline.
   D.   Citalopram and nortriptyline.
   E.   Fluoxetine and paroxetine.

C H A P T E R 2 2

Neuropsychiatric Aspects of Brain Tumors

Select the single best response for each question.

22.1 Which of the following is true regarding the epidemiology of central nervous system (CNS) tumors?

A. The incidence of metastatic brain tumors is twice that of primary brain tumors.
B. Among primary brain tumors, meningiomas are more common than gliomas.
C. The group of gliomas includes both astrocytomas and glioblastomas.
D. Over 90% of brain tumors are located supratentorially.
E. Pituitary adenomas are extremely rare, accounting for less than 2% of brain tumors.

22.2 Demographic variables such as age and sex, as well as concurrent systemic and/or neuropsychiatric disease, may be critical factors in the presentation of CNS tumors. Which of the following is true?

A. In pediatric patients, medulloblastomas are the most common CNS tumor.
B. Gliomas are typically seen in elderly patients.
C. Despite the possibility of CNS tumors being heralded by neuropsychiatric symptoms, primary brain tumors are seen in only a small fraction of psychiatric patients.
D. The most common primary site for metastatic brain tumor is the gastrointestinal tract.
E. Because of their great expanse, the frontal lobes are the site of 40% of all CNS tumors.

22.3 Whereas studies on this topic have lacked precision and controversy remains, specifics of neuropsychiatric symptom presentation may be of some clinical value in the evaluation of the suspected CNS tumor patient. Which of the following is true?

A. Tumors with rapid, aggressive growth are more likely to present with disruptive behavioral and cognitive states, whereas insidiously growing tumors are more likely to present personality changes or mood symptoms.
B. Meningiomas are much more likely to present with psychosis than other tumor histological types, irrespective of neuroanatomical location.
C. Generally, the three most important factors influencing neuropsychiatric symptoms from CNS tumors are tumor histology, neuroanatomical location, and associated neurological signs.
D. Because of the primarily anatomical cause of neuropsychiatric symptoms in CNS tumors, the patient's premorbid psychiatric history is of little relevance.
E. Unilateral CNS tumors are more likely to manifest neuropsychiatric symptoms than are bilateral or multifocal tumors.

22.4 Which of the following is true regarding tumors of the frontal lobes?

A. Tumors of the frontal convexities, called dorsolateral prefrontal syndrome, are associated with "pseudopsychopathic" symptoms, including irritability, lability, and poor social judgment.

B. Orbitofrontal syndrome features apathy, indifference, and psychomotor retardation.

C. Because frontal lobe tumors tend to remain localized, they rarely produce pressure effects and edema.

D. Mood symptoms, including both euphoria and depression, are frequent in frontal lobe tumors.

E. Psychotic symptoms in frontal lobe tumors typically include complex delusions and well-formed hallucinations, largely indistinguishable from symptoms of schizophrenia.

22.5 Which of the following is true regarding tumors of the temporal lobes?

A. Psychotic symptoms in temporal lobe tumors include mood swings and visual, olfactory, and tactile hallucinations in addition to the more typical auditory hallucinations seen in schizophrenia.

B. Temporal lobe tumor patients typically experience affective blunting and social distancing similar to schizophrenic patients.

C. Neuropsychiatric symptoms caused by temporal lobe tumors can easily be differentiated from those of frontal lobe tumors.

D. Temporal lobe tumor patients exhibit personality traits indistinguishable from those of temporal lobe seizure disorder patients.

E. Whereas mood and psychotic symptoms are common in temporal lobe tumor patients, anxiety disorders are rare.

22.6 The clinician must know when to suspect a CNS tumor in a neuropsychiatric patient. All of the following signs or symptoms should lead to increased suspicion of CNS malignancy *except*

A. New onset seizures in an adult.

B. New onset headaches, with increasing frequency and severity.

C. Nausea and vomiting, particularly when associated with headaches.

D. Sensory changes.

E. Generalized neurological signs and symptoms, such as weakness.

22.7 The psychopharmacological management of neuropsychiatric symptoms may be critical in relieving symptoms and restoring function. Which of the following is true regarding the specific considerations of psychopharmacological therapy of CNS tumor patients?

A. Because of the anatomic substrate of psychotic symptoms, full-dose antipsychotic therapy is usually needed.

B. Because they have been rigorously studied and found to be safe in this population, atypical antipsychotic agents are the treatment of choice for psychosis due to CNS tumors.

C. Antiparkinsonian agents potentiate the risk of delirium in brain tumor patients, particularly when combined with low-potency typical antipsychotic agents.

D. Because it lowers the seizure threshold in brain tumor patients, the use of methylphenidate is problematic in these patients.

E. Electroconvulsive therapy (ECT) remains contraindicated in brain tumor patients with mood symptoms.

CHAPTER 23

Neuropsychiatric Aspects of Human Immunodeficiency Virus Infection of the Central Nervous System

Select the single best response for each question.

23.1 Neuropsychiatric illnesses resulting from human immunodeficiency virus (HIV) disease are of major importance to all clinicians working with these patients. Which of the following is true?

A. The most common neuropsychiatric illness in HIV disease is psychotic disorder.
B. Cognitive impairment may present early in the course of HIV disease but is largely unrelated to disease progression.
C. Neuropathological examination of the brains of HIV-infected patients characteristically reveals more dramatic widened sulcal spaces, as opposed to ventricular atrophy.
D. Because HIV dementia is considered a subcortical dementia, histological study of the cortex reveals minimal loss of dendritic area.
E. HIV has been detected in the central nervous system (CNS) within 14 days of infection, supporting a primary role for HIV in neuropsychiatric illness.

23.2 Which of the following pairs are the most common opportunistic CNS infections in HIV?

A. *Toxoplasma gondii* and *Candida albicans*.
B. *Cryptococcus neoformans* and *Candida albicans*.
C. *Aspergillus fumigatus* and *Toxoplasma gondii*.
D. *Cryptococcus neoformans* and *Toxoplasma gondii*.
E. *Candida albicans* and *Aspergillus fumigatus*.

23.3 Cerebrospinal fluid (CSF) studies must be considered in evaluation of mental status changes in patients with HIV disease. Which of the following is true?

A. The amount of CSF virus and antibodies correlate directly with degree of cognitive impairment.
B. CSF β_2-microglobulin is a sensitive marker for dementia severity.
C. CSF homovanillic acid (HVA) is decreased in HIV and directly correlates with severity of dementia.
D. Whereas depressive and anxiety symptoms are common in HIV patients, they have not yet been correlated to CSF immune function markers.
E. Increased levels of quinolinic acid are seen in HIV dementia but not in CNS opportunistic infections in the absence of HIV dementia.

23.4   The specific neurobehavioral assessment of HIV dementia may help classification of HIV-related cognitive symptoms. Which of the following is true?

  A. Symptoms of deficient memory registration, storage, and retrieval and decreased psychomotor speed and motor function are considered cortical symptoms.
  B. Symptoms such as aphasia, agnosia, and apraxia are generally present early in the disease process.
  C. Vague cognitive symptoms of decreased "cognitive efficiency" are seen often in at least 20% of HIV patients during the initial stages of the disease.
  D. Severe HIV dementia is infrequently associated with psychotic symptoms.
  E. Classical frontal-lobe symptoms, such as conceptualization and problem-solving difficulties, are restricted to the late stages of HIV dementia.

23.5   Psychopharmacological interventions are of great importance in HIV disease but are subject to several considerations. Which of the following is true?

  A. Because of the nature of the CNS neuropathology, HIV patients with delirium typically require higher doses of antipsychotic agents than do other delirium patients.
  B. Management of depression is especially crucial because HIV-affected patients have a suicide risk twice that of the general population.
  C. Psychostimulant therapy for depression has been demonstrated to be similarly effective to antidepressants for HIV-associated depression.
  D. Among antidepressants for HIV-associated depression, citalopram, nefazodone, venlafaxine, and mirtazapine are the weakest P450 3A4 inhibitors.
  E. β-Blockers are generally safe for chronic use for anxiety disorders in HIV disease because they do not produce dependence.

CHAPTER 24

Neuropsychiatric Aspects of Rheumatic Disease

Select the single best response for each question.

24.1 Systemic lupus erythematosus (SLE) is considered the prototypical autoimmune disease. Which of the following is true regarding the neuropsychiatric symptoms in SLE?

A. The American College of Rheumatology criteria for neurological disorders include dementia, psychosis, and seizures.
B. Inflammatory cells in the cerebral vessel walls are seen in the majority of cases, implicating central nervous system (CNS) vasculitis as the mechanism for neuropsychiatric symptoms.
C. Lupus commonly presents with primarily neuropsychiatric symptoms.
D. Contemporary studies with systematized methodology have validated that psychosis is common in SLE.
E. Suicidal behavior in SLE has been correlated with active disease and abnormal electroencephalogram (EEG).

24.2 Neuropsychiatric diagnosis in SLE may be challenging because of the multiplicity of symptoms and variably progressive nature of the illness. Which of the following is true?

A. Cognitive deficits (on neuropsychological examination) have been reported in one-half of SLE patients without previous CNS disease.
B. Cognitive impairment in SLE is closely correlated to white matter disease on magnetic resonance imaging (MRI).
C. Cognitive impairment in SLE has been correlated to the presence of antiphospholipid antibody.
D. MRI generally reveals periventricular, rather than subcortical white-matter lesions, which assists in differentiation from multiple sclerosis.
E. MRI findings are rare in SLE patients without CNS symptoms.

24.3 Which of the following is true regarding Sjögren's syndrome?

A. Cortical dementia is a common neuropsychiatric finding.
B. The Minnesota Multiphasic Personality Inventory (MMPI) scales of hypochondriasis, depression, and hysteria have been found to be elevated in patients with Sjögren's syndrome.
C. Whereas parkinsonism is reported in patients with Sjögren's syndrome, it is no more common than in other rheumatic illnesses.
D. MRI reveals white- and gray-matter hyperintensities only in symptomatic patients.
E. Serum antineuronal antibodies may be found but do not correlate to presence or absence of neuropsychiatric symptoms.

24.4 A middle-aged male presents with fever, weight loss, hypertension, fatigue, purpura, ulcers, headache, and livedo reticularis. On examination, psychosis, confusion, and cognitive impairment are noted. A likely diagnosis is

    A. Polyarteritis nodosa.
    B. Takayasu's arteritis.
    C. Giant cell arteritis.
    D. Wegener's granulomatosis.
    E. Churg-Strauss syndrome.

24.5 Corticosteroids are a mainstay of treatment of autoimmune disease but may induce neuropsychiatric symptoms in their own right. Which of the following is true?

    A. Neuropsychiatric syndromes are seen in more than 20% of patients following the use of corticosteroids as an idiosyncratic, rather than dose-dependent, phenomenon.
    B. Neuropsychiatric symptoms occur early in the course of treatment and disappear when treatment is over, without a withdrawal syndrome.
    C. Prior history of mood disorder profoundly increases the risk of corticosteroid-induced mood disorder.
    D. Steroid dementia is a relatively common syndrome among corticosteroid-induced neuropsychiatric syndromes.
    E. Antipsychotic medications should be used to counter corticosteroid-induced psychotic symptoms.

C H A P T E R 2 5

Neuropsychiatric Aspects of Endocrine Disorders

Select the single best response for each question.

25.1 Insulin-dependent diabetes mellitus (IDDM) is in many ways the prototypical metabolic disorder with substantial neuropsychiatric comorbidity. Which of the following is true regarding the neuropsychiatric aspects of diabetes mellitus?

   A. Impaired performance on visuospatial tasks is associated with children who develop diabetes mellitus before the age of 5 years, compared with children with an older age at onset.
   B. Symptomatic hypoglycemia episodes are correlated with abnormal neuropsychological test performance, but asymptomatic hypoglycemia episodes are not.
   C. Degree of chronic metabolic control (based on measurements of glycosylated hemoglobin) has not been correlated to neuropsychological test performance.
   D. The prevalence of depression in diabetes is much higher than in other chronic diseases.
   E. When symptoms of depression that may be attributed to the diabetic condition are excluded from a diagnosis of a mood disorder, the prevalence of depression in diabetic patients is decreased by 50%.

25.2 Management of depression in diabetic patients may be of great importance in facilitating medical compliance and self-care. Which of the following is true regarding management of depression in diabetic patients?

   A. In both IDDM and non-insulin-dependent diabetes mellitus (NIDDM), the diabetic condition predates the onset of depressive symptoms.
   B. A depressed state correlates with increased insulin resistance in some patients.
   C. Depression has been associated with an increased risk of diabetic retinopathy in NIDDM (type II) diabetes but not in IDDM (type I) diabetes.
   D. Because of their risk of increased appetite and blood glucose, tricyclic antidepressants (TCAs) should be avoided in diabetic patients with neuropathic pain.
   E. Despite their tendency to modestly increase serum glucose levels, selective serotonin reuptake inhibitors (SSRIs) are preferred for depressed diabetic patients because of their overall greater safety in these patients.

25.3 Hypothyroidism serves as a model for neuropsychiatric symptoms directly attributable to a metabolic illness. Which of the following is true?

    A. Because of the physical lethargy experienced by hypothyroid patients, anxiety symptoms are rare, in less than 5%.

    B. The most severe cognitive manifestation in hypothyroidism is dementia.

    C. Replacement of thyroid hormone in the form of T_3 (rather than T_4) has a specific effect on improving depressed mood but a negligible effect on cognitive performance.

    D. Mood disorders, typically depression, have been found in 50% of patients with hypothyroidism.

    E. Psychotic symptoms are the second most common group of neuropsychiatric illnesses in unselected hypothyroid populations.

25.4 Because of advances in analysis of thyroid function and greater appreciation of the neuropsychiatric correlates of various thyroid disturbances, a system of grading has been developed. A patient who exhibits elevated thyroid-stimulating hormone (TSH), normal thyroid hormone levels, exaggerated TSH response to thyrotropin-releasing hormone (TRH), and increased risk of major depression that responds poorly to antidepressants would be said to have which grade of hypothyroidism?

    A. Grade I.

    B. Grade II.

    C. Grade III.

    D. Grade IV.

    E. Grade V.

25.5 Hyperthyroidism has also been associated with a specific range of neuropsychiatric symptoms and syndromes. Which of the following is true?

    A. Because of the degree of systemic metabolic disturbances in hyperthyroidism, the majority of patients exhibit psychopathology as a result of hyperthyroidism.

    B. In studies of both selected and unselected hyperthyroidism patients, anxiety disorders are the most common neuropsychiatric illnesses.

    C. Cognitive disturbance in hyperthyroidism is as common as it is in hypothyroidism.

    D. In hyperthyroid patients with depressive symptoms, the physical symptoms of hyperthyroidism precede mood symptoms in the vast majority of cases.

    E. In hyperthyroidism, both mania and psychosis are rare.

25.6 In Cushing's syndrome, which of the following is true regarding neuropsychiatric comorbidity?

    A. Mania, simulating bipolar disorder, is seen as commonly as is depression.

    B. The most common neuropsychiatric presentation in Cushing's syndrome is a mixed profile of anxiety and depression.

    C. Treatment of the hormonal disturbance in Cushing's syndrome rarely reverses mood symptoms without concurrent antidepressants.

    D. Delirium is common in Cushing's syndrome and is the most likely cause of psychotic symptoms.

    E. Cognitive impairment, usually of a moderate degree, is common in Cushing's syndrome.

25.7 Parathyroid disease, although relatively uncommon, has been associated with neuropsychiatric illnesses. Which of the following is true?

A. Neuropsychiatric symptoms tend to be stereotypical irrespective of the serum calcium level.
B. Psychiatric symptoms tend to remain persistent despite parathyroidectomy.
C. Mood disorders are the most common neuropsychiatric disturbance in hypoparathyroidism.
D. The risk and types of neuropsychiatric symptoms in hypoparathyroidism are the same for idiopathic and surgical types.
E. Correction of serum calcium levels in hypoparathyroidism has been found to improve neuropsychiatric symptoms.

CHAPTER 26

Neuropsychiatric Aspects of Poisons and Toxins

Select the single best response for each question.

26.1 Aluminum is a ubiquitous metal with numerous industrial and medical applications. Unfortunately, aluminum poisoning may result in substantial neuropsychiatric pathology. Which of the following is true regarding aluminum poisoning?

A. Aluminum is readily absorbed via the gastrointestinal tract, with intraluminal pH having a negligible role in degree of absorption.

B. Patients with acute renal failure often have a precipitous onset of dialysis encephalopathy, featuring personality changes and psychotic symptoms.

C. Dementia due to aluminum toxicity in dialysis patients characteristically features disturbed concentration, attention, orientation, and memory.

D. Electroencephalographic changes in aluminum-toxicity dementia are only seen after the onset of cognitive symptoms.

E. Despite characteristic electroencephalographic abnormalities, seizures and myoclonic jerks are not typical clinical findings.

26.2 Arsenic is an element associated with many industrial processes. Which of the following is true regarding arsenic poisoning and its neuropsychiatric manifestations?

A. Arsenic localizes in the erythrocytes and platelets but not in leukocytes.

B. Neuropsychiatric manifestations of arsenic poisoning are a direct result of its ability to readily penetrate the blood-brain barrier.

C. Acute exposure to arsenic typically produces visual disturbances.

D. Laboratory methods for arsenic analysis include hair analysis to assess both acute and long-term exposure.

E. Seizures, muscle spasms, and muscular twitching may follow acute exposure.

26.3 Lead and manganese poisoning are associated with characteristic neuropsychiatric symptoms. Which of the following is true?

A. Clinical symptoms of lead poisoning emerge at blood levels of 400 mg/L in both children and adults.

B. The first recognizable symptoms of lead poisoning are headaches, tremor, and seizures.

C. Seizures caused by lead toxicity are generalized, not focal, and respond to antiepileptic medications.

D. Manganese toxicity features a sequence of neuropsychiatric disturbances, progressing from mood and psychotic symptoms, to parkinsonian motor symptoms, and finally to frank dystonias and chorea.

E. Blood and urinary manganese levels correlate well with degree of clinical symptoms.

26.4   Mercury poisoning may be a particularly serious problem in certain high-risk occupations. Which of the following is true regarding mercury poisoning?

A. Elemental mercury is particularly dangerous because it is readily absorbed both by inhalation and ingestion.
B. Organic mercury, such as alkyl mercury, is lipid soluble and profoundly neurotoxic.
C. Exposure to inhaled elemental mercury leads to characteristic neuropsychiatric symptoms such as coarse tremor, increased energy, hypersexuality, and mania.
D. Dentists exposed to organic mercury have been found to have decreased motor speed and visual scanning with preserved concentration, memory, and coordination.
E. Methylmercury poisoning is associated with headache, irritability, and depression, and is treated with British anti-Lewisite (BAL).

26.5   Carbon monoxide poisoning is often encountered in suicide attempts. Which of the following is true regarding the neuropsychiatric implications of carbon monoxide poisoning?

A. Acute exposure to carbon monoxide results in disorientation to time and place but not to person.
B. A brief recovery period following exposure may be followed by cognitive, psychotic, and mood symptoms 2–4 weeks later.
C. The greater affinity of hemoglobin for carbon monoxide than for oxygen (approximately 20 times greater) accounts for the potency of carbon monoxide as a poison.
D. The most common symptoms in the delayed neuropsychiatric syndrome of carbon monoxide poisoning include apathy, disorientation, amnesia, and delusions.
E. The electroencephalogram (EEG) is a valuable predictive test because patients with markedly abnormal EEGs do not recover substantially.

26.6   Which of the following is true regarding neuropsychiatric manifestations of organophosphate intoxication?

A. Organophosphates are environmentally problematic because of their propensity to resist rapid degradation.
B. Mild exposure to organophosphates produces anxiety, restlessness, dry mouth, dryness of the conjunctivae, and pupillary mydriasis.
C. Moderate exposure to organophosphates leads to tremors, depression, tachycardia, hypotonia, and seizures.
D. The onset of symptoms from organophosphate toxicity is rapid (within several minutes), irrespective of route of exposure.
E. Neuropsychiatric symptoms such as depression, fatigue, anxiety, and irritability may persist for 1 year following exposure to organophosphates.

CHAPTER 27

Neuropsychiatric Aspects of Ethanol and Other Chemical Dependencies

Select the single best response for each question.

27.1   The substance-related phenomenon of specific physical and/or behavioral/motivational disturbances that present when a drug is discontinued or reduced in dose is referred to as

   A.   Tolerance.
   B.   Sensitization.
   C.   Reverse tolerance.
   D.   Dependence.
   E.   Withdrawal.

27.2   Which of the following drugs acts by the stimulation of monoamine release?

   A.   Opiates.
   B.   Cocaine.
   C.   Amphetamine.
   D.   Hallucinogens.
   E.   Phencyclidine (PCP).

27.3   The locus coeruleus has been implicated in mechanisms of substance dependence. Which of the following is true?

   A.   Inhibition of the locus coeruleus is the cause of the physical symptoms of opiate withdrawal.
   B.   The acute effects of opiates on locus coeruleus neurons occur via direct effects on the K^+ channel and Na^+ current.
   C.   Tolerance, withdrawal, and dependence are in part mediated by upregulation of the cyclic adenosine monophosphate (cAMP) pathway in locus coeruleus neurons.
   D.   Long-term opiate administration is associated with inhibition of norepinephrine synthesis.
   E.   Administration of glutamate receptor antagonists into the locus coeruleus stimulates its activity in opiate withdrawal.

27.4 Regarding the phenomenon of "priming" in drug abuse (wherein a small reexposure to an abused drug leads to relapse), which of the following is *not* true?

    A. Priming has been demonstrated for both opiates and psychostimulants.

    B. Cross-priming refers to opiates being used to prime relapse into abuse of psychostimulants.

    C. Priming injections of opiates and psychostimulants into the nucleus accumbens (NA) induce relapse into opioid-seeking behavior in animals.

    D. Infusions of opioids into brain regions rich in opioid receptors produce a vigorous increase in drug-seeking behavior.

    E. Dopamine antagonists block the priming effects of opioids and psychostimulants.

27.5 Psychosocial stress is commonly associated with relapse into drug abuse. Which of the following is true?

    A. In animals, stress-induced relapse into heroin-seeking behavior requires physical dependence.

    B. Stress-induced heroin-seeking behavior in animals is fully attenuated by pretreatment with dopamine antagonists.

    C. Stress activates the prefrontal cortex and inhibits the pathway from the frontal cortex to dopamine neurons in the ventral tegmental area (VTA).

    D. Drug-withdrawal states readily induce drug-seeking behavior in animals.

    E. Activation of D_2, D_3, and D_4 receptors in rats induces relapse in cocaine-seeking behavior.

27.6 Various structural changes have been described in the VTA and the NA in response to long-term treatment with morphine, cocaine, or alcohol. Which of the following is *not* true after long-term substance exposure?

    A. Tyrosine hydroxylase levels are increased in the VTA.

    B. Tyrosine hydroxylase levels are decreased in the NA.

    C. Neurofilament levels are decreased in the VTA.

    D. The size of VTA dopamine neurons is decreased.

    E. There is an increase in axoplasmic transport from the VTA to the NA.

CHAPTER 28

Neuropsychiatric Aspects of Dementias Associated With Motor Dysfunction

Select the single best response for each question.

28.1   Which of the following is true regarding dementia due to Huntington's disease?

    A.   Aphasia is prominent.

    B.   Positron emission tomography (PET) studies demonstrate hypometabolism in the caudate nucleus.

    C.   Degeneration begins in the anterior caudate nucleus and proceeds posteriorly.

    D.   Severity of motor symptoms is independent of the emotional state.

    E.   Degeneration of the frontal lobes correlates more closely with deficits in executive functions than does degeneration of the caudate nucleus.

28.2   Specific neuropsychiatric findings (some of which require elucidation by formal neuropsychological examination) of dementia due to Huntington's disease typically include which one of the following?

    A.   Early loss of language functions.

    B.   Greater impairment in recognition than retrieval memory.

    C.   Anomia.

    D.   Defects in planning, organizing, and mental flexibility.

    E.   Lack of awareness of cognitive deficits.

28.3   Which of the following is true regarding dementia due to Parkinson's disease?

    A.   There is a high concordance rate for identical twins, suggesting strong genetic factors.

    B.   Neuronal loss in the nucleus basalis of Meynert is a typical finding in both idiopathic and postencephalitic Parkinson's disease with dementia.

    C.   Because dementia due to Parkinson's disease is a subcortical dementia, visuospatial impairment is rare.

    D.   Executive function deficits are common.

    E.   Communication difficulties in dementia due to Parkinson's disease are caused solely by dysarthria, not language difficulties.

28.4 Which of the following is true regarding the diagnosis and management of noncognitive neuropsychiatric symptoms in dementia due to Parkinson's disease?

A. Mood disorders are more common in late-onset cases.

B. Atypical depression in Parkinson's disease features reversed neurovegetative signs rather than anxiety.

C. Medications are the most common cause of psychotic symptoms in Parkinson's disease.

D. Dopamine agonists and anticholinergics effectively treat postural instability.

E. Selegiline may be safely combined with low-dose selective serotonin reuptake inhibitors (SSRIs) in Parkinson's disease.

28.5 Dementia with Lewy bodies (DLB) is an increasingly appreciated form of dementia, with a characteristic pattern of neuropsychiatric symptoms. Which of the following is true regarding DLB?

A. Visual hallucinations, usually unformed and fleeting, are common early in the course of DLB.

B. Fluctuations in cognitive performance, but not level of consciousness, are characteristic.

C. Depression is less common in DLB than in other types of dementia.

D. Greater frontal lobe atrophy in DLB reliably differentiates DLB from Alzheimer's disease.

E. DLB patients tend to respond as well as or better than Alzheimer's disease patients to cholinesterase inhibitors.

28.6 Which of the following is true regarding progressive supranuclear palsy (PSP)?

A. Smooth pursuit eye movements are affected before saccadic eye movements.

B. Severe dementia early in the illness is typical.

C. Aphasia, apraxia, and agnosia are prominent symptoms.

D. Forced, inappropriate expressions of crying, laughter, or rage are typical.

E. Because of the presence of parkinsonian symptoms in PSP, levodopa treatment is generally successful for motor symptoms.

28.7 Which of the following is true of Fahr's disease?

A. Fahr's disease is a rare, inherited, autosomal recessive disorder.

B. Calcification (evident on neuroimaging) is restricted to the basal ganglia.

C. Patients typically present in early adulthood with dementia in the absence of mood or psychotic symptoms.

D. Apathy and memory impairments are prominent, with spared language functions.

E. Fahr's disease has been associated with hyperparathyroidism.

C H A P T E R   2 9

Neuropsychiatric Aspects of Alzheimer's Disease and Other Dementing Illnesses

Select the single best response for each question.

29.1   Alzheimer's disease (AD) is the most common dementing illness in the United States and is associated with specific neuropathological findings and clinical neuropsychiatric symptoms. Which of the following is true?

    A.   The cortical degeneration in AD typically affects the primary motor and sensory cortex, whereas subcortical structures are spared.

    B.   Genes for amyloid precursor protein, presenilin 1 (PS1), and presenilin 2 (PS2) are all coded on chromosome 21, correlating with the much higher risk of AD in Down syndrome.

    C.   Because the apolipoprotein-E (APOE) ε4 allele is strongly correlated with early onset and more severe AD, it is presently recommended that asymptomatic individuals be screened for this gene.

    D.   The combination of APOE ε4 allele and head injury further increases the risk of subsequent AD.

    E.   Seizures early in the illness strongly suggest a diagnosis of AD.

29.2   Which of the following is true regarding the neuropsychiatric symptoms in AD?

    A.   AD primarily is a diagnosis of exclusion and should be diagnosed presumptively after "reversible" dementias have been ruled out.

    B.   The cortical symptoms of apraxia and agnosia are commonly seen together in the early stages of the disease.

    C.   Verbal fluency and reading aloud by rote are lost early, whereas simple verbal repetition is preserved until late in the clinical course.

    D.   Personality changes are extremely common, and the usual personality manifestation is increased aggressiveness and disinhibition.

    E.   Delusions, including delusions of theft, infidelity, or abandonment, are present in up to 50% of AD patients.

29.3 Which of the following is true regarding the clinical and neuroimaging manifestations of AD?

A. Hallucinations, particularly auditory hallucinations, are seen in 50% of patients.
B. Mood symptoms are common in AD, and 40% of patients meet criteria for a major depressive episode.
C. Because of the risk of comorbid psychotic and depressive disorders, the risk of suicide in AD is high.
D. Studies with positron emission tomography with fluorodeoxyglucose (FDG-PET) reveal early loss of frontal lobe glucose utilization, followed by a later loss in the temporal lobes.
E. Magnetic resonance imaging (MRI) findings of hippocampal atrophy can be a sensitive early marker for AD.

29.4 Frontotemporal dementia (FTD) may come to the psychiatrist's attention because of the propensity for disorganized and/or disruptive behavior. Which of the following is true regarding FTD?

A. Age at onset for FTD is typically greater than 65 years.
B. Memory and visuospatial skills are degraded early, with relative preservation of language skills.
C. Approximately 15% of patients with amyotrophic lateral sclerosis develop FTD.
D. Because of the locus of neuropathology, naming deficits are rare.
E. As with AD, cholinergic neurons are preferentially affected in FTD.

29.5 Vascular dementia is a common dementia syndrome that must often be differentiated from AD. Which of the following is true regarding vascular dementia?

A. Motor symptoms of vascular dementia may include hyperreflexia, extensor plantar responses, and pseudobulbar palsy, whereas gait abnormalities are rare.
B. Speech difficulties in vascular dementia are equally likely to result from aphasia and dysarthria.
C. Because the neuropathology in vascular dementia is primarily subcortical, personality changes are rare.
D. Severity of comorbid depression correlates strongly with degree of cognitive impairment in vascular dementia.
E. MRI is preferable to computed tomography (CT) because of its superiority in imaging subcortical structures.

29.6 Workup for reversible causes of dementia may reveal a correctable cause in up to 15% of patients. All of the following studies are included in a routine dementia assessment *except*

A. Syphilis serology.
B. Complete blood count (CBC).
C. Vitamin B$_{12}$.
D. Thyroid-stimulating hormone (TSH).
E. Serum glucose.

29.7 Dementia due to normal-pressure hydrocephalus (NPH) is potentially reversible. Numerous neuropsychiatric symptoms have been described in association with NPH. Which of the following is *not* typical of NPH?

A. Aphasia, agnosia, and apraxia.
B. Gait disturbance.
C. Visuospatial disturbances.
D. Impaired abstraction.
E. Apathy.

CHAPTER 30

Neuropsychiatric Aspects of Schizophrenia

Select the single best response for each question.

30.1   The symptoms of schizophrenia have been classified as belonging to three major domains: 1) "positive" symptoms such as hallucinations and delusions, 2) thought disorder and bizarre behavior, and 3) "negative" symptoms such as anhedonia and poverty of thought. Which symptom was the most frequently reported psychotic symptom in the 1974 World Health Organization International Pilot Study of Schizophrenia?

   A. Lack of insight.
   B. Auditory hallucinations.
   C. Ideas of reference.
   D. Suspiciousness.
   E. Flatness of affect.

30.2   Numerous putative risk factors for the later expression of schizophrenia have been postulated and subjected to clinical investigation. Which of the following is true?

   A. First-degree relatives of schizophrenic patients have a 15%–20% risk of developing schizophrenia.
   B. Perinatal adverse events have been consistently associated with later development of schizophrenia; these events increase risk by 5%–10%, depending on the study.
   C. One compelling association between perinatal adverse events and the later expression of schizophrenia is the vulnerability of hippocampal pyramidal neurons to hypoxia.
   D. The association between winter birth and later development of schizophrenia is small and has not been consistently replicable.
   E. A monozygotic twin of a schizophrenia patient has a nearly 100% chance of developing schizophrenia, supporting a strong genetic component in the risk of this illness.

30.3   Anatomic and histopathological analyses have offered several compelling insights into the neuropathology of schizophrenia. Which of the following is true?

   A. Magnetic resonance imaging (MRI) studies have revealed decreased volume of the superior temporal gyrus, and this finding has been correlated to the presence of delusions and negative symptoms.
   B. In schizophrenic subjects, cells of the primary limbic structures have been found to have abnormal cell size and cell number but normal gross structure and area.
   C. Basal ganglia enlargement (in the caudate nucleus and putamen) seen in schizophrenia is independent of treatment with antipsychotic medication.

D. The failure of normal neuronal migration during intrauterine development in schizophrenic patients is supported by the finding of excess neurons in lower, rather than superficial, layers of the cortex.

E. Decreased expression of glutamic acid decarboxylase (GAD) mRNA in schizophrenic patients is seen only with cell loss in the prefrontal cortex.

30.4   Which of the following is true regarding neurotransmitters in schizophrenia?

A. The study of neurotransmitters and their metabolites in schizophrenia has greatly elucidated the neuropathology of this illness.

B. Dopamine type 2 (D_2)–family receptor density is increased in the caudate nucleus and putamen of schizophrenic subjects.

C. The recent finding of increased D_4 receptors in schizophrenic subjects is especially compelling in understanding the natural history of schizophrenia, because these receptors are unaffected by antipsychotic medication treatment.

D. Schizophrenic patients show an increased release of dopamine into the synapse during the chronic, but not acute, phases of their illness.

E. Norepinephrine levels are consistently and substantially elevated in schizophrenia, and noradrenergic antagonists decrease psychotic symptoms in these patients.

30.5   Several neuropsychological findings are reported in schizophrenia. Which of the following is true?

A. Identical twin studies have shown that the schizophrenic twin has poorer scores on intelligence, memory, and verbal fluency than the unaffected twin.

B. Likely because of the effects of paranoid cognitions, schizophrenic patients tend to perform well on instruments requiring sustained vigilance and attention.

C. First-degree relatives of schizophrenic patients exhibit a higher frequency of cognitive deficits but only when expressing psychotic symptoms.

D. Among relatives of schizophrenic subjects, the cognitive deficits are most dramatic in those with schizoid personality disorder.

E. The smooth-pursuit eye movement disorder in schizophrenia is only evident during active psychotic episodes.

30.6   The impact of psychopharmacology on schizophrenia is an important clinical consideration. Which of the following is true?

A. There have been demonstrations of increased glucose metabolism in the caudate nucleus and putamen of schizophrenic patients after the administration of atypical antipsychotics, but this effect has not been seen with typical agents.

B. Dopamine agonists reduce dopamine synthesis by directly blocking the availability of precursor molecules.

C. The D_2 family of receptors (including D_2, D_3, and D_4) mediate the effects of antipsychotic agents, with most antipsychotics having activity at only one of these sites.

D. As a model for psychotic illness, ketamine is particularly illustrative because it induces both positive and negative symptoms.

E. Ketamine tends to induce psychotic symptoms idiosyncratic to the individual, which is unusual among psychotomimetic drugs.

CHAPTER 31

Neuropsychiatric Aspects of Mood and Affective Disorders

Select the single best response for each question.

31.1   Several neurochemical abnormalities have been implicated in the genesis and symptomatic expression of mood disorders. Which of the following is true?

   A.   Consistent with a monoamine deficiency hypothesis, plasma norepinephrine is decreased in untreated depression.
   B.   Acute antidepressant treatment increases norepinephrine turnover and neuronal norepinephrine uptake.
   C.   A serotonin deficiency state in depression is supported by the finding of increased 5-hydroxytryptamine (serotonin) type 2 (5-HT$_2$) receptor binding in suicide victims.
   D.   Acute treatment with antidepressants increases serotonin turnover and neuronal serotonin uptake.
   E.   Cerebrospinal fluid (CSF) homovanillic acid and γ-aminobutyric acid (GABA) are both increased in untreated depression.

31.2   Various functional endocrine markers may have clinical implications in mood disorders. Which of the following is true regarding endocrine abnormalities in depression?

   A.   The dexamethasone suppression test is abnormal in the vast majority of cases of depression.
   B.   Depressed, euthyroid patients have nevertheless been shown to have elevated levels of circulating thyroid antibodies.
   C.   Depressed patients have decreased corticotropin-releasing hormone (CRH) in the CSF.
   D.   Corticotropin-releasing factor (CRF) binding in the frontal cortex of suicide victims is typically increased.
   E.   Depressed patients show a prompt and large increase in thyroid-stimulating hormone (TSH) following administration of exogenous thyrotropin-releasing hormone (TRH).

31.3   Clinicians frequently encounter significant sleep complaints in depressed patients. Which of the following is true regarding the clinical and sleep laboratory findings in depressed patients?

   A.   Slow-wave sleep in increased in depression.
   B.   Reduced rapid-eye movement (REM) sleep latency is common in depression and is reversed by antidepressants.
   C.   Sleep deprivation produces greater antidepressant effects if administered in the first half of the sleep period.
   D.   Bipolar patients in a depressed episode also show predictable decreased REM latency.
   E.   In depression, the first REM period is of normal length and subsequent REM periods are lengthened.

31.4 Cognitive complaints and decrements in observed cognitive function are common in depression and may be the source of much of the patient's clinical suffering. Which of the following is true?

   A. Impairment in language, perception, and spatial comprehension are common "primary" cognitive complaints in depression.
   B. Depressed patients with cognitive complaints show similar degrees of functional impairment for both effortful and automatic cognitive tasks.
   C. The pattern of specific memory deficits in depression simulates that seen in cortical, rather than subcortical, dementia.
   D. Comparative studies in the cognitive status of treated patients show that tricyclic antidepressants (TCAs) and selective serotonin reuptake inhibitors (SSRIs) have similar effects on improving cognition.
   E. The elderly patient with depressive pseudodementia may have an increased risk of eventual dementia, even if treatment responsive.

31.5 Several neurologic conditions are associated with high risk for mood disorders and serve as convenient models for the study of neuroanatomic localization in depression. Which of the following is true?

   A. Patients with traumatic brain injury show a high correlation between left-sided lesions and subsequent mood disorders.
   B. Pathological emotions, both laughter and crying, are more common with left-sided lesions.
   C. Positron emission tomography (PET) studies comparing unipolar depression, bipolar depression, and Parkinson's disease with depression have demonstrated that prefrontal, inferior parietal, and anterior cingulate gyrus hypometabolism are seen in all three types of depression.
   D. Depression following lacunar subcortical stroke is associated with bilateral frontal lobe hypometabolism.
   E. Because of the ongoing neuronal degeneration, Parkinson's disease with depression has decreased metabolism in the striatum.

31.6 Which of the following is true regarding functional neuroimaging in primary mood disorders?

   A. Decreased frontal lobe function is the most robust finding in depression.
   B. Although prefrontal activity is common in depression, it does not correlate directly with the degree of clinical symptoms.
   C. Pretreatment hypometabolism in the rostral cingulate predicts response to antidepressant therapy.
   D. Normalization of pretreatment frontal lobe hypometabolism is seen with TCAs and monoamine oxidase inhibitors (MAOIs) but not with SSRIs.
   E. Likely because of the specificity of their effect on serotonin receptors, SSRIs result in downregulation of 5-HT$_{2A}$ receptors, whereas TCAs do not.

C H A P T E R   3 2

Neuropsychiatric Aspects of Anxiety Disorders

Select the single best response for each question.

32.1   Various central nervous system (CNS) lesions and illnesses have been associated with anxiety symptoms and have thus served as models for certain anxiety disorders. Which of the following is true?

   A. Temporal lobe seizures, tumors, lobectomy, and arteriovenous malformations have been associated with panic attacks, with left-sided lesions showing a stronger association than right-sided lesions.
   B. Overlapping mechanisms between temporal lobe seizures have been proposed, but panic disorder is not associated with abnormal electroencephalogram (EEG) and does not respond to antiseizure medication.
   C. The striatal topography hypothesis of basal ganglia lesions held that putamen lesions led to tics, whereas caudate nucleus lesions led to obsessive-compulsive disorder (OCD) symptoms.
   D. Anxiety symptoms are a common neuropsychiatric prodrome in Huntington's disease and lead to generalized anxiety disorder (GAD), but not panic disorder or OCD.
   E. Anxiety symptoms in Alzheimer's disease are most common in the mild stages of illness (Mini-Mental State Exam [MMSE] score of 21–30).

32.2   The common clinical syndromes of stroke and traumatic brain injury (TBI) are an important part of neuropsychiatric practice. In addition to the familiar mood and cognitive symptoms frequently seen in these conditions, anxiety disorders may also cause decreased patient function. Which of the following is true?

   A. Mixed anxiety and depression is more common with left-sided cortical stroke, whereas a "pure" anxiety disorder is more common after right-sided cortical stroke.
   B. Isolated worry is more common with right posterior cerebrovascular accident (CVA), whereas full-spectrum GAD is more common with right anterior CVA.
   C. Poststroke GAD is self-limited, even without treatment, and almost always resolves within 1 year.
   D. Agoraphobia is much less common than GAD after stroke.
   E. Posttraumatic stress disorder (PTSD) after TBI requires early, explicit memory of the traumatizing event.

32.3 OCD is a fascinating and often disabling anxiety disorder that has strong neuroanatomical and neurophysiological implications. Which of the following is true?

A. Clinically effective treatment with a selective serotonin reuptake inhibitor (SSRI) leads to increased cerebrospinal fluid (CSF) 5-hydroxyindoleacetic acid (5-HIAA), suggesting adequate serotonin repletion.

B. Downregulation of serotonin terminal autoreceptors in orbitofrontal cortex follows successful treatment with SSRIs or electroconvulsive therapy (ECT).

C. OCD patients with tics are more likely to respond to SSRIs plus atypical, but not typical, antipsychotics.

D. Reduced caudate nucleus volume has been a consistent finding in OCD.

E. Cortico-striatal-thalamic-cortical (CSTC) activity normalization follows successful OCD treatment with medications or behavioral therapy.

32.4 Panic disorder has also been subject to neuroanatomic and neurophysiological study. Which of the following is true?

A. The dorsal raphe nucleus sends serotonergic projections that stimulate the locus coeruleus.

B. The locus coeruleus sends noradrenergic projections that inhibit the dorsal raphe nucleus.

C. Fluoxetine has been shown to improve panic disorder symptoms; this improvement correlated with a simultaneous decline in a noradrenergic metabolite.

D. Basal ganglia functional abnormalities in panic disorder are as common as in OCD.

E. Panic disorder's clinical responsiveness to benzodiazepines correlates with increased peripheral benzodiazepine binding.

32.5 Though often less dramatic in presentation than OCD or panic disorder, social phobia is a common source of clinical distress. Which of the following is true regarding the neuropsychiatry of social phobia?

A. Although social phobia patients tend to have limited social lives, they are relatively unaffected educationally or vocationally.

B. Enhanced cortisol response in social phobia has been found with fenfluramine, levodopa, and clonidine, suggesting multiple neurochemical pathways.

C. Indirect evidence for a role of dopamine in social phobia includes an association of social phobia with Parkinson's disease and use of antipsychotic medications.

D. Social phobia patients typically have abnormal responses on the dexamethasone suppression test, implicating a hypothalamic-pituitary- adrenal axis abnormality.

E. Treatment of social phobia with SSRIs has been associated with reduced activity in the right temporal cortex.

CHAPTER 33

Neuropsychiatric Disorders of Childhood and Adolescence

Select the single best response for each question.

33.1 Attention-deficit/hyperactivity disorder (ADHD) is a complex neuropsychiatric disorder with onset in childhood and with a variable persistence for years after diagnosis. In addition, neuropsychiatric comorbidity may complicate diagnosis and management. Which of the following is *not* true?

    A. Conduct disorder is seen in 40%–70% of ADHD children.
    B. ADHD is common in pediatric male patients with Tourette's syndrome.
    C. The natural history of ADHD has been estimated to yield spontaneous remission in 30% by adolescence and up to 70% by adulthood.
    D. Boys with ADHD have a stronger family history than do girls, particularly in male relatives.
    E. Low birth weight, fetal alcohol exposure, and lead exposure are common etiological factors.

33.2 An unusual but clinically significant side effect of antipsychotic treatment in children with Tourette's syndrome is

    A. Secondary ADHD.
    B. Phobic anxiety, leading to social phobia.
    C. Major depression.
    D. Neuroleptic malignant syndrome.
    E. Paradoxical visual hallucinations.

33.3 Down syndrome, or trisomy 21, is the most common chromosomal abnormality leading to mental retardation. Because of several central nervous system (CNS) and systemic anomalies, the life expectancy of these patients may be compromised. What is the average life expectancy in patients with Down syndrome?

    A. 35 years.
    B. 40 years.
    C. 50 years.
    D. 55 years.
    E. 60 years.

33.4 Stereotypies are repetitive, apparently purposeless movements such as flicking, twirling, spinning of objects, hand flapping, whirling, and posturing. These movements are characteristic of which neuropsychiatric condition?

A. ADHD.
B. Tourette's syndrome.
C. Conduct disorder.
D. Autism.
E. Down syndrome with mental retardation.

33.5 Seizure disorders are well known for their association with other neuropsychiatric comorbidity. A prominent association has been established between epilepsy, suicidality, and _____, which may be more prominent in temporal lobe epilepsy.

A. Manic episodes.
B. Catatonic posturing.
C. Hyperreligiosity.
D. Learning disabilities.
E. Self-destructive behavior.

33.6 Traumatic brain injury is the cause of more than 25% of hospital admissions in children and is a major source of persistent disability. Which of the following parameters of traumatic brain injury is most strongly related to clinical outcome?

A. Severity of brain injury.
B. Duration of posttraumatic amnesia.
C. Duration of coma.
D. Presence of brainstem injury.
E. Presence of increased intracranial pressure.

C H A P T E R   3 4

Intracellular and Intercellular Principles of Pharmacotherapy for Neuropsychiatric Disorders

Select the single best response for each question.

34.1   Recent research has revealed the increasingly complex and critical roles of glial cells in neuronal function. Which of the following is true regarding this relationship?

   A. Glial cells help maintain the critical balance between excitatory and inhibitory neurotransmitters by recapturing glutamate and γ-aminobutyric acid (GABA) from synapses and then returning them unaltered to their respective neurons.
   B. Glutamate expresses excitotoxicity by the selective opening of sodium channels.
   C. Glial cell line–derived neurotrophic factor (GDNF) has its specific trophic response only on dopamine neurons.
   D. GDNF may ultimately represent a therapeutic intervention for Parkinson's disease and amyotrophic lateral sclerosis.
   E. GDNF's high propensity to penetrate the blood-brain barrier is due to its structure as a short-chain peptide.

34.2   The mechanisms of neurotransmitter synthesis vary among the neurotransmitters that are involved in neuropsychiatric illnesses. Which of the following is true?

   A. The final steps in the synthesis of neurotransmitters, including for neuropeptides, occur in regions proximate to the presynaptic storage site.
   B. Proteins composing the presynaptic voltage-gated calcium channels are physically separated from the proteins devoted to storage vesicle docking and fusion.
   C. Reserpine, as a model for presynaptic neurotransmitter storage disruption, produces a reversible effect on the storage of all biogenic amines.
   D. Presynaptic $GABA_A$ and cholinergic receptors both operate by inducing hyperpolarization.
   E. Presynaptic serotonin receptors, such as 5-hydroxytryptamine type 3 (5-HT_3), admit Ca^{2+} ions and produce depolarization.

34.3 Which of the following statements is true regarding the structure and function of postsynaptic receptors?

A. The most prevalent postsynaptic neuroreceptors form membrane channels or ionophores.
B. Receptors that act at allosteric sites, such as the benzodiazepine receptor, are typically coupled to G proteins.
C. Acetylcholine receptors include nicotinic and muscarinic; of these two types only the nicotinic involves actions of a G protein.
D. Long-term treatment with antidepressants has been shown to downregulate β-adrenergic receptors but not N-methyl-D-aspartate (NMDA) receptors in brain tissue.
E. Serotonin receptors operate via G proteins.

34.4 A drug has been shown to bind to a given postsynaptic receptor but then produce a physiological effect opposite to that produced by a natural neurotransmitter associated with that particular receptor class. This drug is thus acting as a(n)

A. Agonist.
B. Antagonist.
C. Inverse agonist.
D. Partial agonist.
E. Mixed agonist/antagonist.

34.5 Which of the following is true regarding the biochemical structure and/or function of postsynaptic G proteins and second messengers?

A. The G proteins are composed of numerous varieties of α, β, and γ subunits, all of which are interchangeable.
B. The α and γ subunits remain attached to each other and are the moiety that interacts with the neuroreceptor.
C. The action of lithium appears to be by blockade of inositol monophosphate.
D. Inositol triphosphate binds to receptors on the cell membrane and releases intracellular calcium.
E. G protein mechanisms are only seen for excitatory neurotransmitters.

34.6 The study of neurotransmitter/receptor mechanisms is of particular importance in evolving concepts of psychotic illness and in the development of more specific and less neurotoxic antipsychotic medications. Which is true regarding the atypical antipsychotic agents and their specific receptor binding properties?

A. Clozapine has a higher binding affinity for the dopamine D_4 receptor subtype than does haloperidol, accounting for its therapeutic efficacy.
B. The atypical antipsychotics have more 5-HT_{2A} binding affinity than do typical antipsychotics but not necessarily a higher binding affinity for 5-HT_{2A} than the D_2 dopamine receptor.
C. A specific D_4 antagonist was shown to be effective in the treatment of acute psychosis.
D. Haloperidol and atypical antipsychotic agents have similar binding affinity for 5-HT_6 and 5-HT_7 receptors.
E. Despite variations in their binding affinities for D_2 and 5-HT_{2A} receptors, the ratio of 5-HT_{2A} to D_2 binding affinities is similar for clozapine, olanzapine, and risperidone.

C H A P T E R　3 5

Psychopharmacologic Treatments for Patients With Neuropsychiatric Disorders

Select the single best response for each question.

35.1　The general approach to psychopharmacology in neuropsychiatric patients is subject to certain clinical caveats, owing to the implications of neurologic illness on the metabolism and end-organ effects of psychopharmacological agents. Which of the following is true?

A. A poststroke patient with depression and aggression should be treated preferentially with tricyclic antidepressant monotherapy.

B. A brain-injured patient with complex partial seizures comorbid with manic symptoms of labile affect and impulsive behavior should first receive combination therapy with lithium and phenytoin to maximize control of each symptom domain.

C. Because of the increased sensitivity of neuropsychiatric patients to side effects with psychotropic medications, initial and ultimate or final doses should be less than those for other adult patients.

D. Because of the likelihood of cognitive impairment and compliance problems, the psychiatrist should rely on medication blood levels as a marker for medication efficacy.

E. Treatment of psychiatric symptoms before they exacerbate the patient's neurological illness may improve overall functioning (e.g., in multiple sclerosis).

35.2　For clinical purposes, it is useful in neuropsychiatry to group depression, apathy, and deficit states. Which of the following is true regarding these conditions?

A. The use of relatively activating antidepressants should be avoided in anxiously depressed neuropsychiatric patients.

B. Apathy states refer to cognitive and behavioral slowing due to a mood disorder.

C. There is a consistent relationship among many neuropsychiatric illnesses that depression severity predicts more rapid subsequent neurological deterioration and ultimately disability.

D. Postmortem studies of depressed patients with Alzheimer's disease have shown deficits in both the serotonin and norepinephrine pathways.

E. Systemic medications, such as corticosteroids, calcium-channel blockers, and β-blockers, are consistently shown to induce depression when mean differences in treated versus untreated groups are examined.

35.3   Which of the following is true regarding the treatment of depression in neuropsychiatric patients?

A.   Selective serotonin reuptake inhibitors (SSRIs) have a role both in post–cerebrovascular accident depression and in pathological crying in the absence of full-spectrum depression.

B.   Tricyclic antidepressants (TCAs) are as well-tolerated as SSRIs in patients with multiple sclerosis.

C.   A major benefit of SSRIs in neuropsychiatric patients is the absence of risk of extrapyramidal side effects (EPS).

D.   Bupropion is problematic in neuropsychiatric patients because its propensity to induce seizures is idiosyncratic rather than dose dependent.

E.   Methylphenidate may induce euphoric mood in patients with Parkinson's disease.

35.4   Which of the following is true regarding the treatment of depression, apathy, and deficit states in neuropsychiatric illness?

A.   Psychostimulants must be used with caution in patients with brain injury because of a propensity to increase seizure frequency.

B.   Pemoline has been shown to effectively treat fatigue in patients with multiple sclerosis and has been well-tolerated.

C.   Electroconvulsive therapy (ECT) has not been effective in depression due to Huntington's disease because of ECT-induced worsening of movement disorder symptoms.

D.   Parenteral benzodiazepines are a highly effective alternative to ECT in catatonic states.

E.   Catatonia is more likely to be caused by psychotic states than affective disorders.

35.5   Which of the following is true regarding psychosis in the context of neuropsychiatric illness?

A.   Psychosis is common in patients who have had a stroke and who have multiple sclerosis.

B.   Psychosis in human immunodeficiency virus (HIV) dementia, as opposed to Alzheimer's disease, is strongly associated with severe dementia and malignant disease progression.

C.   Psychosis in Parkinson's disease is caused by the degeneration of cortical structures and is not a side effect of antiparkinsonian medications.

D.   Clozapine has been documented as the most effective antipsychotic agent in Parkinson's disease, and low doses are often effective.

E.   In dementia, risperidone 2 mg/day has been demonstrated to have a low risk of EPS.

35.6   Which of the following is true regarding mania and anxiety in neuropsychiatric illness?

A.   Mania in patients with traumatic brain injury is no more common than in the general population.

B.   Patients with multiple sclerosis are more likely to have mania than are populations of general psychiatric inpatients.

C.   Agitation is as common in multi-infarct vascular dementia as in Alzheimer's disease.

D.   Anxious states are common in damage to the right anterior inferior temporal lobe, whereas manic states are less localized.

E.   Serotonergic deficiencies in Alzheimer's disease have been consistently related to behavioral agitation.

35.7 β-Blockers may be a relatively underutilized group of medications for agitated states in neuropsychiatry. Which of the following is true?

A. Placebo-controlled studies show a greater than 50% rate of response.
B. Response is typically manifest within 3 weeks.
C. Anti-agitation effects are due to central, rather than peripheral, effects.
D. Secondary depression induced by β-blockers is relatively common and leads to discontinuation of treatment.
E. The dose of propranolol may need to be as high as 800 mg/day, although lower doses are typical.

C H A P T E R   3 6

Psychotherapy for Patients With Neuropsychiatric Disorders

Select the single best response for each question.

36.1 Psychological defense mechanisms are best conceptualized as existing on a continuum from the most mature (representing the highest level of psychological health), through an intermediate group of less mature, to the most immature (typifying psychotic functioning). Which of the following defenses is classified among the most mature defenses?

A. Suppression.
B. Reaction formation.
C. Rationalization.
D. Displacement.
E. Isolation.

36.2 There have been described a number of misidentification syndromes that may result from neuropsychiatric illness that are manifest in specific patterns of perception and behavior. If a patient perceives that a previously familiar person has now assumed another bodily form, the phenomenon is referred to as

A. Capgras's delusion.
B. Frégoli type misidentification.
C. Metamorphosis.
D. Subjective doubles.
E. Reverse Frégoli type misidentification.

36.3 Psychological functioning in patients with schizophrenia has been offered as an explanatory model for the understanding of psychological functioning of patients with other neuropsychiatric illnesses. All of the following psychological processes are shared between schizophrenic patients and those with neuropsychiatric illnesses *except*

A. Catastrophic reactions to overwhelming stress.
B. Involuntary concreteness.
C. Incapability of moving among different levels of abstraction.
D. Fear of novelty.
E. The use of emotions to overcome cognitive problems.

36.4 Which of the following is true of the psychological functioning of patients with traumatic brain injury?

   A. The patient's family is most disrupted by the patient's cognitive difficulties rather than emotional symptoms.
   B. Psychotherapeutic interventions should be delayed until the emergency of irritable temper, typically at 3 months after injury.
   C. To avoid burnout of treatment team staff, day-long one-on-one rehabilitation is best avoided.
   D. Problem-solving exercises should begin with the concrete and, after mastery, should then proceed to the more abstract.
   E. Posttraumatic headache rarely persists beyond 3 months and thus is unlikely to disrupt psychotherapy at this point.

36.5 Intervention with the patient's family aids in greater functional recovery following traumatic brain injury. Which of the following is true?

   A. Family involvement should begin only after a strong therapeutic alliance with the patient has been established over time.
   B. The psychotherapist should avoid informing the family in great detail about the process of functional recovery, so as to preserve patient privacy.
   C. Family members should be warned about the possibility of being manipulated by the injured patient.
   D. The therapist should avoid a stance of active advocacy for the brain-injured patient in the family situation.
   E. The therapist should guard against the family generalizing the patient's learning to novel situations, focusing instead on the issue at hand only.

36.6 The neuropsychiatrist may be called upon to treat the unfortunate victim of paralyzing spinal cord injury. Which of the following is true regarding the psychological and psychotherapeutic aspects of spinal cord injury?

   A. Clinically significant major depression is seen in the majority of patients within 6 months of injury.
   B. Cognitive-behavioral interventions for spinal cord injury patients have been associated with fewer readmissions and higher levels of adjustment.
   C. An internal locus of control predicts depression 2 years after injury.
   D. Because of the high risk of depression, cognitive-behavioral therapy should routinely be offered to all victims of spinal cord injury.
   E. Because of the demographics of those affected by spinal cord injury, individual and group psychotherapy should focus on introspection and avoid action orientation.

36.7 Parkinson's disease is a neurodegenerative disorder with notable psychiatric comorbidity. Which of the following is true regarding the psychotherapeutic issues involved in Parkinson's disease?

   A. To assist the patient's process of acceptance of his or her illness, early use of support groups (including more advanced patients) is advised.
   B. Behavioral interventions for parkinsonian gait include focus on straightening posture, attention to balance, and renormalizing the arm swing.
   C. The psychotherapist must be attuned to the presence of violent and threatening hallucinosis in 30% of patients treated with L-dopa.
   D. Greater degrees of gait disturbance, tremor, and postural abnormalities reliably predict cognitive impairment.
   E. As with other neurodegenerative diseases, communication in Parkinson's disease is compromised by language impairments.

36.8 Multiple sclerosis is another major chronic illness of the central nervous system that will come to the attention of the psychiatrist. Which of the following is true of the psychological and psychotherapeutic aspects of multiple sclerosis?

   A. Paradoxical serenity (pleasant affect despite neurologic impairments) is more common early in the illness.
   B. The chronic and unpredictable nature of multiple sclerosis may lead to excess dependence on physicians.
   C. Despite the possibility of functional losses of frontal lobe function, the patient should be challenged to undertake significant reordering of defenses when symptomatic.
   D. The psychotherapist should limit theoretical and practical approaches to supportive psychotherapy models only.
   E. Dementia in multiple sclerosis affects memory encoding and storage more than retrieval.

C H A P T E R   3 7

Cognitive Rehabilitation and Behavior Therapy for Patients With Neuropsychiatric Disorders

Select the single best response for each question.

37.1   The general approach of the clinician to the cognitive rehabilitation of the neuropsychiatric patient establishes the therapeutic context of the clinical goals. Which of the following is true?

   A. In cognitive rehabilitation after stroke, reorganization of motor skills is possible for only the first year after the stroke.
   B. Cognitive rehabilitation of the traumatic brain injured patient is likely to focus on a specific cognitive deficit rather than general approaches to memory and attentional disturbances.
   C. Because of cognitive deficits, anger management training is unlikely to benefit the traumatic brain injury patient.
   D. Psychostimulant medication may facilitate rehabilitation in patients with frontal lobe injuries.
   E. Psychological recovery in traumatic brain injury is usually greater for ecologically relevant behaviors than on performance on standardized tests.

37.2   Several instrumental models using computers to facilitate cognitive rehabilitation have been developed. Which of the following is *not* an area of training in the Orientation Remedial model of Ben-Yishay and associates (Ben-Yishay and Diller 1981)?

   A. Attending and reacting to environmental signals.
   B. Timing responses to changing environmental cues.
   C. Practice of active vigilance.
   D. Time estimation.
   E. Synchronization of response to simple, repetitive rhythms.

37.3   A cognitively impaired patient is instructed to enhance his or her memory function by constructing a story from newly presented material to facilitate encoding. This is an example of

   A. Semantic elaboration.
   B. Face-name association.
   C. Peg mnemonics.
   D. Method of loci.
   E. Direct retraining.

37.4 Which of the following is true regarding visual-perceptual disorders and the approaches to cognitive rehabilitation?

A. Visual-perceptual deficits are most common after left-sided occipital stroke.
B. Hemispatial neglect syndrome is most often experienced in the right hemispace.
C. A light board with colored lights and a fixed target is used for visual scanning training.
D. Visual scanning training as a sole cognitive intervention was found to improve visual-perceptual functioning in brain-injured patients when compared with those patients who were treated with standard occupational therapy.
E. Hemispatial neglect is most common in right-hemisphere stroke.

37.5 There may be spatial localization of neuropsychiatric symptoms following injury to the cortex that affects the cognitive rehabilitation of patients. Which of the following behavioral symptoms is more commonly a sequel of temporal, rather than frontal, lobe injury?

A. Paranoid ideation.
B. Social disinhibition.
C. Reduced attention.
D. Distractibility.
E. Affective lability.

37.6 In a behavioral treatment paradigm, the behavioral therapist has noted a reliable relationship between a specific target behavior and an environmental consequence. The therapist removes the environmental consequence, and the target behavior thereafter is reduced to a near-zero rate of occurrence. This phenomenon is called

A. Positive reinforcement.
B. Negative reinforcement.
C. Punishment.
D. Antecedent.
E. Extinction.

CHAPTER 38

Ethical and Legal Issues in Neuropsychiatry

Select the single best response for each question.

38.1 The legal concept of *competency* has a substantial impact on neuropsychiatric practice, particularly in those patients presenting with cognitive impairments. Which of the following is true?

A. The definition, requirements, and application of the term *competency* vary widely, depending on the issue at hand.

B. Capacity refers to an individual's abilities with regard to display of intact cognitive and decision-making function in a wide range of acts.

C. A mentally ill patient can be held to be incompetent based entirely on the evaluation of a clinician.

D. Institutionalization for mental illness results in the patient being assumed to be incompetent.

E. All minors are assumed to be incompetent.

38.2 The neuropsychiatrist may be called upon to comment on a patient's ability to give informed consent for or to refuse a proposed medical/surgical procedure. All of the following standards apply to this determination *except*

A. Communication of a choice.

B. Demonstration of understanding of information provided.

C. Appreciation one's current situation and the relative risks and benefits of treatment options.

D. Absence of a cognitive disorder on standardized examination.

E. Rationality in the decision-making process.

38.3 When the patient is deficient in the capacity to make medical decisions, a proxy decision maker may be needed. There are several alternatives provided for in the law. Which of the following surrogate choices may be excluded from decisions regarding the treatment of mental disorders?

A. Court-appointed guardian.

B. Treatment review panel.

C. Substituted consent of the court.

D. Institutional administrator or committee.

E. Proxy consent of next of kin.

38.4 The "right to die" may lead to psychiatric evaluation and need for opinion. Which is true regarding the legal status of this issue?

A. The *Cruzan* decision held that the state did not have the right to maintain the patient's life against the family's wishes.
B. The Court distinguished between food and water on the one hand and mechanical ventilation on the other.
C. Physicians are now strongly encouraged to seek clear and competent instructions regarding future treatment decisions, such as with a living will.
D. The right to decline life-sustaining treatment is absolute.
E. As a result of the *Cruzan* decision, physicians will not be held liable for overtreatment of critically ill patients.

38.5 Which is true regarding the insanity defense in criminal proceedings?

A. This defense requires that the accused is incompetent to stand trial.
B. The insanity defense is estimated to be successful in only 10% of the times it is attempted.
C. The estimated rate of not guilty by reason of insanity is estimated at less than 1% of all felony arrests.
D. The Comprehensive Crime Control Act of 1984 supports the volitional prong of the insanity defense.
E. Mental retardation is not an adequate basis for the insanity defense; only Axis I illnesses are allowed.

C H A P T E R   3 9

Educational and Certification Issues in Neuropsychiatry

Select the single best response for each question.

39.1   The requirement for clinical experience in neurology in psychiatry residency programs in the United States has been specified by the Accreditation Council on Graduate Medical Education (ACGME) since 1987. How many months of neurology experience are presently required?

   A. 1 month.
   B. 2 months.
   C. 3 months.
   D. 4 months.
   E. 6 months.

39.2   The 2001 revision of ACGME Essentials for Training in General Psychiatry includes all of the following requirements *except*

   A. Diagnosis and treatment of neurologic disorders encountered in psychiatric practice.
   B. Indications for and limitations of common neuropsychological tests.
   C. Systemic instruction in neurobiology.
   D. Performance and recording of neurological examination.
   E. Interpretation of electroencephalograms (EEGs).

39.3   Combined training in psychiatry and neurology has been proposed as an educational pathway for neuropsychiatrists. Which of the following is true?

   A. Combined training requires a minimum of 5 years.
   B. The first postgraduate year requires 6 months of internal medicine and 3 months each of neurology and psychiatry.
   C. A minimum of 2 years must be spent each in psychiatry and neurology.
   D. All U.S. combined residencies are currently accredited.
   E. Dual training leads to dual board eligibility and dual hospital privileges.

CHAPTER 1

Cellular and Molecular Biology of the Neuron

Select the single best response for each question.

1.1   In the central nervous system (CNS), both chemical and electrical synapses are critical for neural activity. Regarding chemically mediated synapses and their neurotransmitters, which of the following is true?

   A.   Chemical synapses are faster than electrical synapses.
   B.   Chemical synapses are limited in utility because they do not allow for signal amplification.
   C.   Chemical synapses can modulate the activity of other cells through activation of second-messenger cascades.
   D.   Small molecule transmitters (e.g., glutamate, γ-aminobutyric acid [GABA], and glycine) are stored in large, dense-core vesicles.
   E.   Neuropeptides (e.g., somatostatin, endorphins, and enkephalins) mediate fast synaptic transmission.

The correct response is option C.

Most CNS synaptic connections are mediated by chemical neurotransmitters. Although chemical synapses are slower than electrical ones, they allow for signal amplification, may be inhibitory as well as excitatory, are susceptible to a wide range of modulation, and can modulate the activities of other cells through the release of transmitters activating second-messenger cascades. **(p. 9)**

1.2   GABA receptors are ubiquitous in the CNS and have different conformational and neurophysiological properties. Regarding these receptors, which of the following is true?

   A. $GABA_A$ receptors are metabotropic receptors.
   B.   The $GABA_A$ receptor-channel complex is composed of five subunits.
   C. $GABA_B$ receptors are primarily located postsynaptically.
   D.   Clinical actions of benzodiazepines and barbiturates are proportional to their binding potential at $GABA_B$ receptors.
   E.   Benzodiazepines increase GABA current by increasing the amount of "open" time in receptor channels.

The correct response is option B.

$GABA_A$ receptors are members of the nicotinic acetylcholine receptor superfamily. The $GABA_A$ receptor-channel complex is composed of five subunits from α, β, γ, and ρ families. This gives rise to receptors with varying properties. Because most of the subunits have multiple subtypes, there is a potential for an extraordinary diversity of $GABA_A$ receptor function. **(pp. 14–15)**

1.3 The generation of long-term potentiation (LTP) is critical in the neurophysiology of memory. In the mechanism of the generation of LTP in the mammalian hippocampus, which of the following is true?

A. LTP results from the coincident activation of α-amino-3-hydroxy-5-methylisoxazole-4-propionic acid (AMPA) receptors and postsynaptic hyperpolarization.

B. LTP requires Ca^{2+} efflux from postsynaptic neurons.

C. "Silent" synapses contain only AMPA receptors before induction of LTP and can be activated by insertion of new N-methyl-D-aspartate (NMDA) receptors.

D. LTP is composed of early and late phases, both of which require induction of new protein synthesis.

E. LTP and long-term depression (LTD) function in a dynamic equilibrium to maintain memory.

The correct response is option E.

LTP and LTD function dynamically to eliminate irrelevant memories and to fine-tune lasting ones.

LTP activates sufficient numbers of AMPA receptors to cause a significant postsynaptic depolarization. NMDA receptors facilitate Ca^{2+} influx into the postsynaptic dendritic spine. "Silent" synapses contain NMDA receptors before induction of LTP and can be activated by stimulation-dependent insertion of new AMPA receptors. LTP is composed of early and late phases. Early LTP requires protein synthesis, whereas late LTP requires both new transcription and translation. **(pp. 19–22)**

1.4 In neuronal development and modulation, the neuron develops following a specific sequence of steps. Which of the following is the correct order for neuronal growth?

A. Determination, proliferation, migration, axonal elongation, synapse formation, synapse refinement, cell death.

B. Determination, migration, proliferation, axonal elongation, synapse formation, synapse refinement, cell death.

C. Determination, axonal elongation, proliferation, migration, synapse formation, synapse refinement, cell death.

D. Proliferation, determination, migration, axonal elongation, synapse formation, synapse refinement, cell death.

E. Proliferation, determination, axonal elongation, migration, synapse refinement, synapse formation, cell death.

The correct response is option A.

The correct order for neuronal development is determination, proliferation, migration, axonal elongation, synapse formation, synapse refinement, cell death. **(p. 22, Figure 1–14)**

1.5 In neuronal migration, neurons migrate from the "inside out" to reach their final spatial destinations within a laminar structure. What is the laminar organization of neuronal zones, from pial surface to the ventricles?

A. Marginal zone, cortical plate, subplate, intermediate zone, subventricular zone, ventricular zone.

B. Marginal zone, cortical plate, subplate, intermediate zone, ventricular zone, subventricular zone.

C. Cortical plate, subplate, marginal zone, intermediate zone, subventricular zone, ventricular zone.

D. Cortical plate, marginal zone, subplate, intermediate zone, ventricular zone, subventricular zone.

E. Marginal zone, cortical plate, subplate, ventricular zone, intermediate zone, subventricular zone.

The correct response is option A.

Laminar organization is shown diagrammatically in Figure 1–15, with the order (from pial to ventricular surface): marginal zone, cortical plate, subplate, intermediate zone, subventricular zone, and ventricular zone. **(p. 25)**

1.6   In the stages of neuronal maturation, the final stage is often apoptosis. The process of apoptosis is characterized by all of the following properties *except*

   A. It is a genetically programmed form of cell death.
   B. It occurs to cells deprived of neurotrophic fibers.
   C. Cytoplasmic shrinkage occurs.
   D. Ribonucleic acid (RNA) and protein synthesis is required for this process.
   E. An inflammatory response is triggered.

The correct response is option E.

Apoptosis, a genetically programmed form of cell death, is characterized by cytoplasmic shrinkage, RNA and protein synthesis, chromatin condensation, and degradation of deoxyribonucleic acid (DNA) into oligonucleosomal fragments. Unlike necrosis, apoptosis does not trigger an inflammatory response. **(p. 29)**

1.7   Several clinical neuropsychiatric disorders can be linked to specific neuroanatomic loci and/or particular neuropathological processes. Regarding the neuropathology of various neuropsychiatric disorders, which of the following is true?

   A. Striatal degeneration in Huntington's disease is linked to underproduction of a critical synaptic vesicle–associated protein.
   B. A delayed result of a viral infection may be causative in some cases of Parkinson's disease.
   C. 1-Methyl-4-phenyl-1,2,3,6-tetrahydropyridine (MPTP) may produce Parkinson's disease by receptor occupancy and blockade, rather than a neurotoxic mechanism.
   D. Parkinson's disease may also be caused by pathological excess of neurotrophic factors.
   E. Alzheimer's disease features loss of basal forebrain cholinergic neurons, which may follow an excess of or aberrant handling of nerve growth factor.

The correct response is option B.

In Parkinson's disease, a selective loss of dopaminergic neurons in the substantia nigra may be the delayed result of a viral process.

   Striatal degeneration in Huntington's disease appears to be caused by the overproduction of a synaptic vesicle–associated protein that may translate into NMDA receptor–mediated excitotoxicity. In Parkinson's disease, a loss of dopaminergic neurons in the substantia nigra may be the result of a neurotoxic mechanism or a deficiency in the neurotrophic factors. In Alzheimer's disease, the loss of cholinergic neurons may result from a deficiency or aberrant handling of nerve growth factor. **(p. 34)**

C H A P T E R 2

Human Electrophysiology and Basic Sleep Mechanisms

Select the single best response for each question.

2.1 The electroencephalogram (EEG) features tracings of brain activity that are classified in frequency bands, which correlate with different central nervous system (CNS) actions. Which of the following is true regarding EEG frequency bands?

A. Delta waves (4–8 Hz) are associated with rapid eye movement (REM) sleep.

B. Alpha waves (8–14 Hz) are best recorded over the parietal region.

C. Alpha rhythm occurs during wakefulness, generally appearing on eye closure and vanishing on eye opening.

D. The genesis of alpha rhythms has been established to be in the thalamus.

E. Beta and gamma bands occur over nonoverlapping frequency ranges greater than 14 Hz.

The correct response is option C.

The alpha rhythm has a frequency range of 8–14 Hz and is best recorded over the occipital scalp region. It occurs during wakefulness, usually appearing on eye closure and disappearing with eye opening. **(pp. 44–45)**

2.2 Sleep is characterized by a sequence of sleep stages with specific EEG and behavioral correlates. In sleep studies, which of the following is true?

A. The typical polysomnogram consists of simultaneous monitoring of the EEG, electromyogram (EMG), and electro-oculogram (EOG).

B. Stage I sleep is characterized by the emergence of 14–16 Hz sleep spindles.

C. Stages III and IV sleep feature (respectively) greater and lesser occurrence of 0.5–4 Hz delta waves.

D. As the sleep period progresses, the subject spends less time in REM sleep with successive sleep cycles.

E. It is more difficult to arouse a subject from REM sleep than from Stage IV sleep.

The correct response is option A.

A typical study of sleep includes recordings of the EEG, of muscle tone (the EMG), and of eye movements (the EOG). This is known as a *polysomnogram*, and the recording process is called *polysomnography*.

Stage I sleep is characterized by low-voltage, high-frequency EEG patterns and slow, rolling eye movements. Stages III and IV are characterized, respectively, by lesser and greater occurrence of slow delta waves. It is easier to arouse a subject from REM sleep than from Stage IV sleep. **(pp. 45–47)**

2.3 Sleep patterns (both on EEG and in sleep behavior) change predictably across the life span. Regarding the change in sleep architecture over time, which of the following is true?

A. Infants sleep one-half of the time, with REM sleep occupying one-half of total sleep time.
B. The percentage of REM sleep declines rapidly throughout childhood, and the adult percentage of REM sleep is reached by age 20 years.
C. Adults spend approximately 35% of total sleep time in REM.
D. Non-REM (NREM) sleep (Stages III and IV) is minimal in newborns.
E. NREM sleep reaches a maximum by age 20 years before subsequently declining.

The correct response is option D.

NREM sleep (Stages III and IV) is minimal in newborns but increases during the first years of life, reaching a maximum at about age 10 years and declining thereafter.

Infants sleep two-thirds of the time, with REM sleep occupying one-half of total sleep time. Adults spend approximately 20% of total sleep time in REM. **(p. 47)**

2.4 CNS activity as recorded by the EEG has been localized to various arousal mechanisms. Regarding the neurophysiology of EEG activation, which of the following is true?

A. Brainstem cholinergic nuclei (laterodorsal and pedunculopontine tegmental nuclei, LDT/PPT) have high discharge rates only in waking, with low discharge rates in REM and slow-wave sleep (SWS).
B. EEG synchronization refers to the EEG of wakefulness.
C. Brainstem reticular neuronal projections, using inhibitory amino acid neurotransmission, also participate in EEG activation.
D. Locus coeruleus and dorsal raphe nucleus monoaminergic neurons are active in REM sleep.
E. Projections from the basal forebrain nucleus basalis of Meynert play an important role in EEG activation.

The correct response is option E.

In addition to brainstem cholinergic systems, cholinergic and noncholinergic input to cortex and to thalamus from the basal forebrain cholinergic nucleus basalis of Meynert plays an important role in EEG activation.

Brainstem cholinergic nuclei have high discharge rates in waking and REM sleep and low discharge rates in SWS. *EEG desynchronization* refers to the EEG of wakefulness. Brainstem reticular neuronal projections, using excitatory amino acid neurotransmission, participate in EEG activation. Locus coeruleus and dorsal raphe nucleus monoaminergic neurons are silent in REM sleep. **(p. 49)**

2.5 Adenosine has been demonstrated to have specific roles in sleep physiology. Regarding the role of adenosine in sleep, which of the following is true?

A. Adenosine's role mediating sleepiness following prolonged wakefulness appears to be mediated by excitation of basal forebrain neurons.
B. Stimulant beverages (e.g., coffee, tea) increase alertness by an agonist effect on adenosine receptors.
C. Increased metabolism leads to an increase in extracellular adenosine in the basal forebrain.
D. Basal forebrain extracellular adenosine levels decrease with prolonged wakefulness.
E. With prolonged wakefulness, adenosine levels change uniformly in various brain regions important to behavioral state control.

The correct response is option C.

Increased metabolism leads to reduced high-energy phospate stores and increased extracellular adenosine in the basal forebrain.

Adenosine appears to be a mediator of the sleepiness following prolonged wakefulness, a role in which its inhibitory action may be especially important. Coffee and tea increase alertness by an antagonist effect on adenosine receptors. Basal forebrain extracellular adenosine levels increase with prolonged wakefulness. Adenosine levels in other brain regions are affected in different ways with prolonged wakefulness. **(pp. 53–55)**

2.6   Acetylcholine has been found to have important roles in sleep structure. Regarding cholinergic mechanisms in REM sleep, which of the following is true?

   A. Injection of acetylcholine agonists into the pontine reticular formation produces a REM-like state by activation of primarily nicotinic receptors.
   B. Approximately 50% of reticular formation neurons are excited by cholinergic agonists, primarily via nicotinic receptor effects.
   C. Cholinergic neurons are critical in the production of the low-voltage, fast EEG pattern in REM sleep and upon awakening.
   D. Electrical stimulation of the LDT decreases REM sleep.
   E. Cholinergic neurons may be critical in producing hyperpolarization of reticular effector neurons for REM sleep events.

The correct response is option C.

Cholinergic neurons are important in the production of the low-voltage, fast EEG patterns in both REM sleep and waking.

Injection of compounds that are acetylcholine agonists into the pontine reticular formation produces a REM-like state by activation of muscarinic receptors. In vitro studies show that a majority (80%) of reticular formation neurons are excited by cholinergic agonists, with muscarinic effects being especially pronounced. Electrical stimulation of the LDT increases REM sleep. Cholinergic neurons may be critical in producing depolarization of reticular effector neurons for REM sleep events. **(p. 57)**

2.7   Narcolepsy is a sleep disorder that causes significant disruption in patients' lives. Regarding narcolepsy, all of the following are true *except*

   A. It is a chronic sleep disorder.
   B. Patients experience excessive daytime sleepiness.
   C. Recent research shows undetectable levels of the neuropeptide orexin in narcolepsy patients.
   D. Delayed onset of REM is typical.
   E. Hypnagogic hallucinations are common.

The correct response is option D.

Narcolepsy is a chronic sleep disorder characterized by excessive daytime sleepiness, fragmented sleep, and other symptoms (such as hypnagogic hallucinations and sleep-onset REM periods, and sleep paralysis) that are indicative of abnormal REM sleep expression. **(pp. 62–63)**

C H A P T E R   3

Functional Neuroanatomy: Neuropsychological Correlates of Cortical and Subcortical Damage

Select the single best response for each question.

3.1   Cortical localization of specific functions can be conceptualized on both a "right-left" dichotomy and an "anterior-posterior" one. Regarding lateral and longitudinal specialization of cortical functions, which of the following statements is true?

A. Less than 50% of left-handed persons are left-brain dominant for language functions.
B. Whereas the majority of the population process spoken and written language with the left hemisphere, languages derived from visuogestural signals (e.g., American Sign Language) are primarily processed in the right hemisphere.
C. In most subjects, the right hemisphere processes nonverbal information, such as complex visual patterns and nonverbal auditory information.
D. Posterior regions of the brain are primarily responsible for the execution of motor behavior.
E. Prosodic expression is a right-hemisphere function localized in the anatomical counterpart to Wernicke's area in the left hemisphere.

The correct response is option C.

The right hemisphere processes nonverbal information such as faces and music. The left hemisphere processes language in 98% of right-handed individuals and in 70% of left-handed individuals, and this is true for auditory languages as well as visuogestural signals (e.g., American Sign Language).

Posterior regions of the brain are dedicated to sensation and perception. Prosodic expression is a right-hemisphere function; the right frontal operculum is a counterpart to Broca's area in the left hemisphere. **(pp. 73–74)**

3.2   The hippocampal complex is a critical structure of the mesial temporal region of the temporal lobes. Which of the following statements about the hippocampal complex (structure and/or function) is true?

A. Anatomically, the hippocampal complex includes the hippocampus and amygdala.
B. The left hippocampal complex subserves the acquisition of new verbal material, and the right hippocampal complex is responsible for the acquisition of novel nonverbal material.
C. The hippocampal complexes are equally responsible for the acquisition of declarative and nondeclarative memory.

D. Patients with Alzheimer's disease with hippocampal damage exhibit marked impairment of both anterograde memory and the learning of novel perceptuomotor skills.

E. The hippocampal complex is a principal storage repository for "old" memories.

The correct response is option B.

There are two hippocampal complexes, one in the left and one in the right hemisphere. The left has verbal specialization and the right, nonverbal.

The hippocampal complex includes the hippocampus and the adjacent entorhinal and perirhinal cortices. The hippocampal system does not appear to have a role in the acquisition of nondeclarative memory. Patients with Alzheimer's disease with hippocampal damage exhibit marked impairment of anterograde memory but intact learning of nondeclarative information such as new perceptuomotor skills. The hippocampal system is not the principal repository for old memories. **(pp. 75–79)**

3.3 Perceptual and communication functions involve several complementary cortical functions, all of which must be integrated for normal perception of the environment and use of language. Regarding the functions of lexical retrieval ("naming") and visual recognition, which of the following statements is true?

A. Lexical retrieval is localized in the inferotemporal region of the temporal lobe, sparing the temporal pole.

B. Lesions in the temporal lobe that impair lexical retrieval typically impair other language functions such as grammar, syntax, and repetition.

C. Damage to the right anterolateral temporal region has been reported to cause a defect in naming of facial expressions.

D. The occipitotemporal junction consists of the posterior part of the inferotemporal region plus the superior portions of Brodmann's areas 17, 18, and 19.

E. Prosopagnosia, the inability to recognize previously known faces, is usually accompanied by an inability to recognize gender and age from face information.

The correct response is option C.

Lesions of the right anterolateral temporal region have been reported to cause a selective defect in naming facial expressions, such as fear or happiness.

Structures in the anterior and inferolateral left temporal lobe play a key role in lexical retrieval. Lesions in the temporal lobe do not typically cause defects in grammar, syntax, phonetic implementation, and repetition. The occipitotemporal junction consists of the posterior part of the inferotemporal region plus the inferior portion of Brodmann's areas 18 and 19. Prosopagnosia is characterized by an inability to recognize previously known faces and learn new ones while the ability to judge gender and estimate age from face information is well preserved. **(pp. 80–82)**

3.4 Balint's syndrome is a devastating "central" disorder of visually related behaviors. Which of the following is true regarding Balint's syndrome?

A. It is caused by a lesion of the ventral component of the occipital cortex.

B. The lesion affects the primary visual cortex but spares the visual association cortices.

C. Balint's syndrome can only be produced with bilateral occipital lesions.

D. The three cardinal clinical features are visual disorientation, ocular apraxia, and optic ataxia.

E. Ocular apraxia refers to a disturbance in visually guided reaching behavior (e.g., accurately pointing at a target object using visual guidance).

The correct response is option D.

Balint's syndrome is generally caused by bilateral lesions in the superior occipital region, although a right lesion can also produce the syndrome. The three principal clinical features of Balint's syndrome are visual disorientation (or simultanagnosia), ocular apraxia (or psychic gaze paralysis), and optic ataxia.

Ocular apraxia is a deficit of visual scanning, while optic apraxia is a disturbance of visually guided reaching. **(pp. 85–86)**

3.5   The occipital lobes are exclusively devoted to processing visual information. Regarding the neuropsychological consequences of various occipital lesions, which of the following is true?

   A.   Acquired achromatopsia involves variable parts of the visual field and is typically associated with impairment in form vision.
   B.   Acquired achromatopsia is associated with impairment in the naming of colors.
   C.   A patient with a unilateral left occipitotemporal lesion may have right hemiachromatopsia but will rarely have an associated alexia.
   D.   Patients with apperceptive visual agnosia will have difficulty in producing the image of a whole entity when given just a part of a visual stimulus (e.g., they cannot imagine a car as the source of a wheel when presented with the image of a wheel).
   E.   Patients with pure alexia cannot read whole sentences but can always read single words or letters.

The correct response is option D.

Patients with apperceptive visual agnosia fail many standard neuropsychological tests of visual perception, such as matching pieces to form a whole object.

Acquired achromatopsia is a disorder of color perception with preservation of form vision, which is not associated with the inability to name colors. A lesion on the left occipitotemporal region will produce right hemiachromatopsia and also alexia. Patients with pure alexia are unable to read most words and sentences, and, in severe cases, even single letters. **(pp. 87–89)**

3.6   The parietal lobes are crucial for language, mathematical, and recognition functions. Regarding neuropsychological deficits from parietal lobe lesions, which of the following is true?

   A.   Wernicke's aphasia is characterized by fluent paraphasic speech and defective aural comprehension but preserved simple repetition.
   B.   Conduction aphasia is associated with profoundly defective verbatim repetition, nonfluent speech, and impaired reading comprehension.
   C.   Lesions to the inferior parietal lobule may lead to acalculia, an acquired inability to perform simple mathematical calculations.
   D.   Neglect syndromes from right-sided inferior parietal lobule lesions are confined to neglect of intrapersonal space.
   E.   Anosognosia refers to the patient's lack of concern with (rather than lack of recognition of) a neurological and/or neuropsychological deficit.

The correct response is option C.

Left-sided lesions in the inferior parietal lobule may lead to acalculia, wherein patients lose the ability to perform simple mathematical calculations and may even be unable to read or write numbers.

Wernicke's aphasia is characterized by fluent, paraphasic speech, impaired repetition, and defective aural comprehension. Conduction aphasia is associated with marked defects in verbatim repetition, fluent speech, and mildly compromised comprehension. Neglect can involve intrapersonal as well as extrapersonal space. Neglect of intrapersonal space is illustrated by the patient failing to use or denying the existence of the contralateral extremity, even when there is no motor impairment. Neglect of extrapersonal space is illustrated by the patient failing to attend to "external" stimuli, e.g., external objects in the left visual field. Anosognosia is a true recognition defect in which the patient is unaware of acquired motor, sensory, or cognitive deficits. **(pp. 90–94)**

3.7   The frontal lobes are responsible for a wide array of behaviors, ranging from simple interpersonal communication to memory to interpersonal conduct. Which of the following statements is true regarding the neuropsychological correlates of frontal lobe dysfunction?

A. Akinetic mutism may follow lesions to the superior mesial aspect of the frontal lobe.
B. The patient with akinetic mutism makes no effort to communicate by any modality and will not track moving targets with smooth pursuit eye movements.
C. Akinetic mutism is typically more severe with right- as opposed to left-sided lesions.
D. Lesions to the basal forebrain may cause an amnestic syndrome characterized by an absence of confabulation.
E. Lesions to the ventromedial frontal lobe may cause the condition of acquired sociopathy, which is typically associated with an amnestic syndrome and diffuse conventional neuropsychological deficits.

The correct response is option A.

The superior mesial aspect of the frontal lobes is crucial in the initiation of movement and emotional expression. Lesions in this region cause akinetic mutism, a syndrome in which the patient does not communicate, either verbally or by gesture, and maintains a noncommunicative facial expression. Movements are limited to tracking of moving targets.

There does not appear to be a significant difference in the profile of akinetic mutism as a function of the side of the lesion. Patients with ventromedial frontal lobe damage develop a severe disruption of social conduct, a condition termed *acquired sociopathy*. This condition does not provoke memory disturbances, and the patients are free of conventional neuropsychological defects. **(pp. 95–102)**

C H A P T E R   4

Nervous, Endocrine, and Immune System Interactions in Psychiatry

Select the single best response for each question.

4.1 The immune system is characterized by a complex series of cells, proteins, and functional systems. Regarding the basic organization of the immune system, which of the following is true?

A. All immune cells are derived from hematopoietic stem cells, which are located both in the bone marrow and in the peripheral circulation.

B. The two developmental pathways for stem cells are the myeloid line (leading to B cells, T cells, and natural killer [NK] cells) and the lymphoid line (leading to monocytes and granulocytes).

C. Cytokines are soluble immune signaling factors solely responsible for the regulation of cell movement.

D. "Proinflammatory cytokines" include interleukin (IL)-1, interleukin-6, and tumor necrosis factor-alpha and are produced primarily by mast cells

E. Type I interferons (IFNs), IFN-α and IFN-β, have both immunostimulatory and antiproliferative effects.

The correct response is option E.

Type I interferons, a class of cytokine released early during immune response, have antiviral, immunostimulatory, and antiproliferative effects. As such, they are used to treat viral infections (e.g., hepatitis C) and malignant disorders.

All immune cells originate from hematopoietic stem cells in the bone marrow. The myeloid cell line includes monocytes and granulocytes (e.g., neutrophils, basophils, and eosinophils). The lymphoid cell line includes B cells, T cells, and NK cells. Cytokines are soluble immune signaling factors that have systemic effects on a wide range of body functions not limited to the immune system. Proinflammatory cytokines are produced primarily by monocytes and macrophages. **(p. 116)**

4.2 Natural and acquired immunity serve complementary functions through different mechanisms. Regarding the mechanisms and immunological roles of natural and acquired immunity, which of the following statements is true?

A. Innate, or "natural" immunity is primarily mediated by phagocytes (e.g., monocytes and basophils) and NK cells.

B. The acute phase response involves the production of acute phase reactants by the peripheral tissues to isolate invading pathogens.

C. The complement system, acting through a cascade of proteins, is an important part of acquired immunity.

D. The four sequential phases of acquired immunity are induction, activation, effector, and memory.

E. T cell–mediated immunity is referred to as humoral immunity because this immunity can be transferred by cell-free blood products.

The correct response is option D.

Acquired immunity occurs in four conceptually distinct phases: an induction phase, in which an infectious agent or antigen is detected; an activation phase, in which immune cells proliferate and mobilize; an effector phase, in which the agent or antigen is neutralized and eliminated; and a memory phase, in which immune cells capable of responding to reexposure to antigen are maintained in the circulation.

Examples of phagocytes are monocytes and neutrophils. The acute phase response occurs when the liver produces proteins called *acute phase reactants* that help isolate and destroy invading pathogens, control damage to self tissues, and stimulate repair pathways (Baumann and Gauldie 1994). The complement system is an important part of natural immunity. B cell immunity is termed *humoral immunity.* **(pp. 116–121)**

4.3   Stress and immune response have been examined in human subjects in several naturalistic settings. Which of the following statements is true?

A. Elderly caregivers of spouses with Alzheimer's disease have been shown to exhibit decreased lymphocyte proliferation and IL-2 production and a decreased ratio of T-suppressor to T-helper cells.
B. Immunologic effects of long-term stress have included decreased white blood cells, increased peripheral blood lymphocytes, and a decreased ratio of T-helper to T-suppressor cells.
C. In long-term naturalistic stressor studies, nonsocial stressors tend to have a greater immunological effect than social stressors.
D. Spousal caregivers of dementia patients have been found to have impaired wound healing when compared with matched control subjects.
E. Medical students facing examinations and spousal caregivers of Alzheimer's disease patients have been found to have decreased antibody responses to hepatitis A and influenza vaccines.

The correct response is option D.

Immunologic changes associated with stress may have implications for health and disease, as suggested by a study of caregivers of dementia patients with impaired wound healing.

Elderly caregivers of spouses with Alzheimer's disease have been found to exhibit decreased lymphocyte proliferation and IL-2 production, decreased ratio of T-helper to T-suppressor cells (Pariante et al. 1997), and decreased NK cell activity (Esterling et al. 1996). Immunologic effects of long-term stress include increased white blood cells, decreased peripheral blood lymphocytes, decreased cytotoxic/suppressor T cells, and increased antibody titers to herpes simplex virus type I and Epstein-Barr virus. Social (interpersonal) stressors appear to have more profound effects than nonsocial ones. Decreased antibody responses to hepatitis B and influenza vaccines, respectively, have been found in medical students experiencing acute examination stress (Glaser et al. 1992) and spousal caregivers of Alzheimer's disease patients (Kiecolt-Glaser et al. 1996). **(p. 124)**

4.4 The relationship between cancer and psychological stressors has been examined. Which of the following is true?

A. A large Danish study found an increase in cancer, allergic disease, and autoimmune disease in parents whose child was diagnosed with cancer.

B. Major depression has been consistently found to increase the risk of a subsequent new diagnosis of cancer.

C. Research data suggests that psychological variables have a greater impact on the *course* of cancer rather than dramatically increasing its *incidence* risk.

D. Studies of clinical psychiatric interventions in cancer patients (e.g., cognitive-behavioral therapy and group therapy) have consistently found an increase in cancer longevity for patients receiving psychiatric treatments.

E. Studies of psychiatric interventions for cancer patients have generally been targeted to patients at higher risk for psychiatric illness.

The correct response is option C.

Data suggests that psychological factors may have a greater effect once cancer is diagnosed.

A large Danish study (Johansen and Olsen 1997) found no association between the diagnosis of cancer in one's child and an increased odds ratio for the development of cancer, allergies, or autoimmune disease during a period ranging from 7 to 49 years after the child's cancer diagnosis. Not all studies of clinical psychiatric interventions in cancer patients have resulted in consistent findings of increased longevity. In addition, these limited studies have included all patients, not simply those who might be psychiatrically vulnerable to stress-related immune alterations. **(pp. 125–126)**

4.5 Immune function has been studied in patients with depression. Which of the following is true?

A. Peripheral blood findings in depressed patients have included increased lymphocytes, decreased neutrophils, and decreased NK cell activity.

B. A syndrome of "sickness behavior" mimicking major depression follows administration of IFN-α and IL-2.

C. Cerebrospinal fluid (CSF) studies of depressed patients have demonstrated increased levels of IL-6 and soluble IL-6 receptors and decreased levels of IL-1-β.

D. Female patients with depression are more likely to exhibit NK cell decreases than male patients.

E. Decreased acute phase proteins have been found in depressed patients.

The correct response is option B.

A syndrome of "sickness behavior" resembling major depression occurs with the administration of cytokine therapies such as IFN-α and IL-2 (Dantzer et al. 1999). Prominent features of sickness behavior include depressed mood, anhedonia, sleep and appetite disturbances, malaise, and poor concentration.

Peripheral blood findings in depressed patients have included decreased lymphocyte number, increased neutrophil number, and decreased NK cell activity. CSF studies of depressed patients have demonstrated decreased levels of IL-6 and soluble IL-6 receptor and increased levels of IL-1-β. Male patients with depression are more likely to exhibit NK cell decreases than are female patients. Increased acute phase proteins have been found in depressed patients. **(pp. 129–131)**

4.6   Immunologic function in schizophrenia has revealed which one of the following?

A. Peripheral blood findings in schizophrenic patients include decreased B cells, CD4+ lymphocytes, and monocytes.
B. Decreased acute phase proteins have been reported.
C. Increased CD5+ cells have been found, suggesting an autoimmune mechanism in schizophrenia.
D. CSF findings in schizophrenic patients include decreased IL-2 and soluble IL-6 receptors.
E. Increased IL-2 levels in schizophrenia are specific for an autoimmune, rather than infectious, mechanism in the genesis of schizophrenia.

The correct response is option C.

Increased numbers of CD5+ cells have been found, thus suggesting the presence of an autoimmune mechanism in schizophrenia. **(p. 131, Table 4–6)**

References

Dantzer R, Aubert A, Bluthe RM, et al: Mechanisms of the behavioural effects of cytokines. Adv Exp Med Biol 461:83–106, 1999

Esterling BA, Kiecolt-Glaser JK, Glaser R: Psychosocial modulation of cytokine-induced natural killer cell activity in older adults. Psychosom Med 58:264–272, 1996

Glaser R, Kiecolt-Glaser JK, Bonneau RH, et al: Stress-induced modulation of the immune response to recombinant hepatitis B vaccine. Psychosom Med 54:22–29, 1992

Johansen C, Olsen JH: Psychological stress, cancer incidence and mortality from non-malignant diseases. Br J Cancer 75:144–148, 1997

Kiecolt-Glaser JK, Glaser R, Gravenstein S, et al: Chronic stress alters the immune response to influenza virus vaccine in older adults. Proc Natl Acad Sci U S A 93:3043–3047, 1996

Pariante CM, Carpiniello B, Orru MG, et al: Chronic caregiving stress alters peripheral blood immune parameters: the role of age and severity of stress. Psychother Psychosom 66:199–207, 1997

CHAPTER 5

Bedside Neuropsychiatry: Eliciting the Clinical Phenomena of Neuropsychiatric Illness

Select the single best response for each question.

5.1   The clinical examination of the neuropsychiatric patient involves thorough data gathering and specific interviewing strategies. Which of the following statements is true regarding the history and/or examination of a neuropsychiatric patient?

   A.   When questioning a head-injured patient, the duration of loss of consciousness or coma is considered the best indicator for severity of traumatic brain injury.
   B.   Assessment of the length of posttraumatic amnesia should be discerned only by questioning the patient because hospital records are generally unreliable.
   C.   A loss of capacity for divided attention is more suggestive of "functional" psychiatric illness than cerebral disease or injury.
   D.   Regarding observations of dream activity in traumatic brain injury, loss of dream material is specific for left, rather than right, parietal lobe injury.
   E.   Abnormal oral/feeding behavior, such as mouthing and consumption of nonfood items suggests Klüver-Bucy syndrome (bilateral amygdalar disease).

   The correct response is option E.

   Abnormal eating behavior is found in neuropsychiatric patients affected by hyperphagia of hypothalamic disease (where food is irresistible), by Klüver-Bucy syndrome, or by frontal disease.
       Posttraumatic amnesia is the best indicator of severity of traumatic brain injury. The length of anterograde amnesia can be learned either from the patient or from hospital records. A loss of capacity for divided attention is highly indicative of mild cerebral disease. Loss of dream activity occurs with parietal lesions in either hemisphere and with deep bifrontal injury. **(pp. 155–157)**

5.2   Minor physical anomalies may offer a clue to the interpretation of neuropsychiatric syndromes. Regarding the content and application of the Waldrop scale of minor physical anomalies as pertains to neuropsychiatry, which of the following is true?

   A.   The items on this scale are limited to abnormalities of the head and neck.
   B.   Minor physical abnormalities specified are not found in normal individuals and reliably identify neuropsychiatric illness.
   C.   Deviant physical development of the head occurs from the fourth to sixth months of fetal life.
   D.   Minor physical anomalies are associated with schizophrenia, including late-onset schizophrenia.
   E.   Dysmorphic features can readily classify the type of syndrome responsible for mental retardation.

The correct response is option D.

Minor physical abnormalities of the head, hands, and feet are associated with schizophrenia (including late-onset), mood disorder, tardive dyskinesia, autism, schizotypal personality disorder, violent delinquency in boys, inhibited behavior in girls, and violent behavior in criminals.

The Waldrop scale anomalies may occur in healthy individuals, and no individual anomaly, except perhaps abnormal head circumference, has a correlation with psychopathology. The deviant development of the head can be traced to the first 4 months of fetal life. Dysmorphic features in a mentally retarded patient should lead to investigations to identify the cause of the retardation (Ryan and Sunada 1997). **(p. 157)**

5.3   Assessment of eye movements may assist neuropsychiatric diagnosis. Regarding eye movements in neuropsychiatry, which of the following is true?

A. It is generally advisable for the clinician to make inferential descriptions ("Patient was looking at source of hallucinated voices") rather than phenomenological descriptions ("Patient suddenly looked to his left several times in mid-sentence").
B. Stevens's studies and subsequent laboratory studies of eye movement disorders in schizophrenia have addressed saccadic movements.
C. Failure of voluntary lateral gaze is a hallmark of progressive supranuclear palsy.
D. Visual grasping refers to the inability to suppress reflex saccadic eye movements and is seen in schizophrenia.
E. Eye movement disorders, such as slowed saccades and an inability to make a saccadic eye movement without simultaneous head movements, are uncommon in Huntington's disease.

The correct response is option D.

The inability to inhibit reflexive saccades to a target is characteristic of frontal disease and is seen in schizophrenia.

Clinicians' descriptions of eye movements should be phenomenological rather than inferential. Failure of voluntary downgaze is a hallmark of progressive supranuclear palsy but is not always present early in the course (Collins et al. 1995). Slowed saccades, inability to make a saccade without moving the head or blinking, and other eye movement abnormalities are common in Huntington's disease (Leigh et al. 1983). **(pp. 158–159)**

5.4   Speech disorders are relatively common in neuropsychiatric illness. Regarding clinical abnormalities of speech, which of the following is true?

A. In pseudobulbar palsy, slow, strained, and slurred speech are only infrequently accompanied by dysphagia, drooling, and disturbed emotional expression.
B. Acquired stuttering may follow stroke, psychotropic drug ingestion, and extrapyramidal disease.
C. Developmental and acquired stuttering are both characterized by involuntary movements of the face and head, reminiscent of dystonias.
D. Aprosodia (the emotional analog of aphasia) is produced solely by right-sided hemispheric lesions.
E. Echolalia refers to a simple "parroting back" of the examiner's speech by the patient, with no modifications of content or grammar.

The correct response is option B.

Acquired stuttering is unusual but can be caused by stroke, traumatic brain injury, psychotropic drugs, and extrapyramidal disease.

In pseudobulbar palsy, slow, strained, and slurred speech is often accompanied by dysphagia, drooling, and disturbed emotional expression. In developmental but not acquired stuttering, involuntary movements of the face and head resemble those of cranial dystonia. Aprosodia is produced by lesions of either the left or the right hemisphere. Patients with echolalia can make grammatical corrections and content changes when parroting back words, thus demonstrating intact syntactic capabilities. (pp. 160–162)

5.5   The movement disorders in Huntington's disease and tardive dyskinesia can appear to overlap in some patients. Which of the following movement types is more common in Huntington's disease rather than in tardive dyskinesia?

A. Repetitive stereotypic movements.
B. Oro-buccal-lingual site abnormal movements.
C. Improvement of facial dyskinesias with tongue protrusion.
D. Postural instability.
E. Marching in place.

The correct response is option D.

Huntington's disease is characterized by postural instability, bizarre ataxic gait, milkmaid grip, dysarthria, facial dyspraxia, oculomotor disturbances, and head thrusts. (p. 165, Table 5–2)

5.6   Various reflexes can be elicited in the neuropsychiatric patient. Regarding the use of primitive reflexes in clinical examination, which of the following is true?

A. All primitive reflexes reflect underlying neuropathology.
B. The grasp, snout, and palmomental reflexes can be elicited with careful examination in the majority of schizophrenia patients.
C. Primitive reflexes in demented patients predict more cognitive impairment for a given level of functional impairment but do not predict prognosis.
D. They are more common in vascular dementia localized in the frontal lobe than in frontotemporal dementia.
E. The grasp reflex is associated with dysfunction of the supplementary motor area.

The correct response is option E.

The grasp reflex is associated with damage to the supplementary motor area; when the damage is more extensive in the medial frontal cortex, a grope reflex may appear (Hashimoto and Tanaka 1998).

Primitive reflexes may be of clinical significance in specific circumstances. Chen et al. (1995) found infrequently the grasp, snout, and palmomental signs in schizophrenic patients but found them significantly more often than in healthy control subjects. Primitive reflexes in demented patients may be associated with poorer functional capacity and indicate poor prognosis (Molloy et al. 1991; Mölsä et al. 1995). They are commonly present in patients with cerebrovascular disease (Rao et al. 1999), but they may be more common in frontotemporal dementia than in comparably severe vascular dementia with frontal predominance (Sjögren et al. 1997). (pp. 167–168)

5.7　　Orientation and memory are basic parts of the clinical examination of the neuropsychiatric patient. Regarding tests of orientation and memory, which of the following is true?

A. The majority of delirium patients are disoriented for person, place, and time.
B. The delirium patient mistakes the "familiar for the unfamiliar," whereas the schizophrenic patient mistakes the "unfamiliar for the familiar."
C. In attention testing, the insertion of a single number in "forward" order in the backward counting test ("20, 19, 18, 17, 18") is rarely significant.
D. Neglect following a right-hemisphere stroke is usually a permanent deficit.
E. Improved recall with semantic cueing is common in frontal-subcortical dementia.

The correct response is option E.

The improvement of verbal recall with semantic cues implies a disorder of retrieval mechanisms, such as in frontal-subcortical disease (Yuspeh et al. 1998).

The delirious patient mistakes the unfamiliar for the familiar, whereas the schizophrenic patient mistakes the familiar for the unfamiliar. Concentration can be assessed by the patient's capacity to recite the numbers from 20 to 1 in reverse order. Neglect is a transient feature after right-hemisphere stroke, usually disappearing after a few months (Hier et al. 1983). **(pp. 170–171)**

5.8　　Thought disorders in the neuropsychiatric patient are best distinguished as disorders of form and content. In assessment of disorders of form and content of thought in the neuropsychiatric patient, which of the following is true?

A. Confabulation, the fabrication of false "factual" material by the patient, may be either spontaneous or in response to physician inquiries and is exclusively seen in amnestic disorders.
B. The Ganser state, or *Vorbeireden (Vorbeigehen)*, is a syndrome of approximate answers that is caused by a focal cerebral lesion.
C. The Charles Bonnet syndrome is characterized by visual hallucinations without other neuropsychiatric findings and is often accompanied by visual deficits.
D. Vividly colored but unformed visual hallucinations are typical with disease of the upper brainstem and/or thalamus.
E. Pathological laughter and crying are discordant with the enduring emotional state but are only elicited by an emotion-laden stimulus such as seeing strong affective expression in another person.

The correct response is option C.

Visual hallucinations are common in idiopathic schizophrenia. In the elderly, visual hallucinations without other psychopathology, especially with ocular disease with visual loss, are indications of Charles Bonnet syndrome. Patients are generally aware of the unreality of their visions.

Confabulations may be either in response to the examiner's queries or spontaneous, but they are not seen exclusively in amnesia. *Vorbeireden (Vorbeigehen)*, the symptom of approximate answers, is the defining feature of the Ganser state. Whether this symptom rests on organic foundations has been controversial from the outset. Vivid, elaborate, and well-formed visual hallucinations may occur with disease in the upper brainstem or thalamus (Kölmel 1991). Pathological laughter and crying are defined not only by the patient's lack of congruent inner experience but also by their elicitation through nonemotional stimuli. **(pp. 174–176)**

References

Chen EYH, Shapleske J, Luque R, et al: The Cambridge Neurological Inventory: a clinical instrument for assessment of soft neurological signs in psychiatric patients. Psychiatry Res 56:183–204, 1995

Collins SJ, Ahlskog JE, Parisi JE, et al: Progressive supranuclear palsy: neuropathologically based diagnostic clinical criteria. J Neurol Neurosurg Psychiatry 58:167–173, 1995

Hashimoto R, Tanaka Y: Contribution of the supplementary motor area and anterior cingulate gyrus to pathological grasping phenomena. Eur Neurol 40:151–158, 1998

Hier DB, Mondlock J, Caplan LR: Recovery of behavioral abnormalities after right hemisphere stroke. Neurology 33:345–350, 1983

Kölmel HW: Peduncular hallucinations. J Neurol 238:457–459, 1991

Leigh RJ, Newman SA, Folstein SE, et al: Abnormal ocular motor control in Huntington's disease. Neurology 33:1268–1275, 1983

Molloy DW, Clarnette RM, McIlroy WE, et al: Clinical significance of primitive reflexes in Alzheimer's disease. J Am Geriatr Soc 39:1160–1163, 1991

Mölsä PK, Marrila RJ, Rinne UK: Long-term survival and predictors of mortality in Alzheimer's disease and multi-infarct dementia. Acta Neurol Scand 91:159–164, 1995

Rao R, Jackson S, Howard R: Primitive reflexes in cerebrovascular disease: a community study of older people with stroke and carotid stenosis. Int J Geriatr Psychiatry 14:964–972, 1999

Ryan R, Sunada K: Medical evaluation of persons with mental retardation referred for psychiatric assessment. Gen Hosp Psychiatry 19:274–280, 1997

Sjögren M, Wallin A, Edman A: Symptomatological characteristics distinguish between frontotemporal dementia and vascular dementia with a dominant frontal lobe syndrome. Int J Geriatr Psychiatry 12:656–661, 1997

Yuspeh RL, Vanderploeg RD, Kershaw DA: Validity of a semantically cued recall procedure for the Mini-Mental State Examination. Neuropsychiatry Neuropsychol Behav Neurol 11:207–211, 1998

CHAPTER 6

Electrodiagnostic Techniques in Neuropsychiatry

Select the single best response for each question.

6.1   The electroencephalogram (EEG) may be a valuable diagnostic test in neuropsychiatry, particularly in enigmatic cases or obscure clinical presentations. Which of the following statements is true?

A.   The EEG itself is likely to lead to a precise diagnosis in the majority of cases because of highly specific abnormalities on surface electrode tracings.
B.   Disorders affecting deep brain structures or characterized by slow, indolent neuronal damage will typically affect electroencephalographic tracings.
C.   Delirium is associated with generalized slowing and irregular high-voltage beta activity.
D.   Dementia is associated with paroxysmal bifrontal delta activity and asymmetry between cerebral hemispheres.
E.   Benzodiazepine intoxication features characteristic background slowing with the superimposition of alpha, but not beta, frequencies.

The correct response is option D.

The EEG is also a nonspecific indicator of cerebral function. However, certain EEG patterns have been correlated with neuropsychiatric disorders. Dementia is associated with paroxysmal bifrontal delta activity and asymmetry between hemispheres. EEG findings associated with other neuropsychiatric disorders include (Fenton 1989) the following:

- Epilepsy—focal and generalized spikes, sharp waves, polyspikes, and spike-wave complexes
- Delirium—generalized slowing and irregular high-voltage delta activity
- Encephalitis—background slowing, diffuse epileptiform activity, and periodic lateralized epileptiform discharges (PLEDs)
- Barbiturate or benzodiazepine intoxication—background slowing and diffuse superimposed beta activity
- Tumor or infarction—focal slowing at border of infarction or tumor; necrotic tissue is electrically silent
- Aging—generalized slowing of alpha rhythm, diffuse theta and delta activity, decline of low-voltage beta activity, and focal delta activity in temporal areas
- Creutzfeldt-Jakob disease and subacute sclerosing panencephalitis—periodic complexes
- Uremic or hepatic encephalopathy—triphasic waves **(pp. 200–202, Table 6–2)**

6.2   The P300 potential may be affected by certain neuropsychiatric illnesses. Which of the following is true?

A. Schizophrenic patients typically have increased P300 amplitude.
B. Abnormal P300 potentials in schizophrenia are specific to medication-naive patients, because antipsychotic medication normalizes the P300 potentials in patients with schizophrenia.
C. Among personality-disordered patients, borderline personality disorder has been found to have more P300 potential abnormalities.
D. Prolonged P300 latency, a common finding in normal aging, is blunted in schizophrenia.
E. P300 potential abnormalities in schizophrenia appear to be unrelated to cognitive deficits.

The correct response is option C.

P300 abnormalities are more prevalent in patients with borderline personality disorder than in those with other personality disorders. These abnormalities, however, are indistinguishable from those of schizophrenic patients.

Schizophrenic patients have a reduction in P300 amplitude. Abnormalities are evident in both medicated and drug-free patients and are associated with negative symptoms. O'Donnell et al. (1995) reported that prolongation of P300 latency, which is normally associated with aging, is exaggerated in schizophrenic subjects. P300 abnormalities in schizophrenia have been linked to deficits in cognition. **(p. 203)**

6.3   The EEG is most specific for evaluation of seizure disorders. Which of the following is true?

A. Epilepsy has a prevalence in the general population of approximately 0.5%.
B. "Spikes" and "sharp waves" in the electroencephalographic tracings of epileptic patients are rarely associated with "polyspikes" and rarely followed by slow waves.
C. Interictal electroencephalographic abnormalities are rare in epilepsy.
D. "Epileptiform" activity on EEG is present in 25%–30% of the normal population.
E. Epileptiform electroencephalographic tracings are relatively common in schizophrenia but much less so in major depression with psychotic features.

The correct response is option A.

Epilepsy is found in approximately 0.3%–0.6% of adults in the general population.

Spikes, sharp waves, and polyspikes, frequently followed by a slow wave, are often seen interictally in epileptic patients (Aminoff 1986; Goodin and Aminoff 1984). Epileptiform activity is found in 1%–10% of the nonepileptic general population (Zivin et al. 1968). Epileptiform electroencephalographic variants are seen in approximately 30% of patients with schizophrenia and psychotic mood disorders (Inui et al. 1998). **(p. 206)**

6.4   The EEG may reveal abnormalities in the cognitive disorders as well as in normal senescence. Which of the following is true?

A. Background alpha rhythm diminishes steadily between young adulthood and old age.
B. Low-voltage beta activity increases steadily throughout life unless there is the emergence of dementia.
C. Mild diffuse slowing is found in the majority of patients over age 75 years.
D. Electroencephalographic slowing has been correlated with cognitive impairment in dementia but is not related to the number of senile plaques seen neuropathologically.
E. Patients with histologically proven Alzheimer's disease have a nearly 100% risk of abnormal EEG.

The correct response is option E.

Robinson et al. (1994) reported that 92% of subjects with Alzheimer's disease, confirmed prospectively by histopathology, had abnormal electroencephalograms, in contrast to 35% of age-matched control subjects.

The changes in background alpha rhythm vary little with normal aging (Visser 1985). Low-voltage beta activity increases in adults up to age 60 years and declines thereafter. Mild diffuse slowing is found in approximately 20% of healthy elders over age 75. Electroencephalographic slowing has been found to be correlated with the severity of dementia (Fenton 1986) and the number of senile plaques (Deisenhammer and Jellinger 1974) in Alzheimer's disease. **(p. 206)**

6.5 Schizophrenia has been studied with regard to associated electroencephalographic anomalies. Which of the following statements is true regarding the EEG and schizophrenia?

A. Although electroencephalographic abnormalities in schizophrenia are more common than in normal healthy subjects, a characteristic "schizophrenic EEG" has not been described.
B. Numerous studies with adequate control subjects have consistently shown a rate of 80% for abnormal EEG in schizophrenia.
C. Schizophrenic patients have a greatly increased risk of seizure disorder, likely correlating with their greater risk of abnormal EEGs.
D. When electroencephalographic hemispheric asymmetries have been seen in schizophrenic patients, the right hemisphere is generally implicated.
E. A strong family history of schizophrenia predicts an abnormal EEG in a schizophrenic patient.

The correct response is option A.

Although there are no specific electroencephalographic findings in schizophrenia, most studies do show that these patients have more abnormalities than are found in healthy control subjects. Abnormal EEGs have been described in up to 80% of schizophrenic patients, but some studies have reported much lower rates.

Middle-age schizophrenic subjects do not appear to have more clinical seizures than age-matched control subjects (Gelisse et al. 1999). Several studies have documented electroencephalographic asymmetries, particularly in the left hemisphere. The lack of a family history of schizophrenia is associated with an increased likelihood of abnormal electroencephalographic activity in schizophrenic patients. **(p. 206)**

References

Aminoff MJ: Electroencephalography: general principles and clinical applications, in Electrodiagnosis in Clinical Neurology. Edited by Aminoff MJ. New York, Churchill Livingstone, 1986, pp 21–75

Deisenhammer E, Jellinger K: EEG in senile dementia. Electroencephalogr Clin Neurophysiol 36:91, 1974

Fenton GW: The electrophysiology of Alzheimer's disease. Br Med Bull 42:29–33, 1986

Fenton GW: The EEG in neuropsychiatry, in The Bridge Between Neurology and Psychiatry. Edited by Reynolds EH, Trimble MR. Edinburgh, UK, Churchill Livingstone, 1989, pp 302–333

Gelisse P, Samuelian JC, Genton P: Is schizophrenia a risk factor for epilepsy or acute symptomatic seizures? Epilepsia 40(11):1566–1571, 1999

Goodin DS, Aminoff MJ: Does the interictal EEG have a role in the diagnosis of epilepsy? Lancet 1:837–839, 1984

Inui K, Motomura E, Okushima R, et al: Electroencephalographic findings in patients with DSM-IV mood disorder, schizophrenia, and other psychotic disorders. Biol Psychiatry 43(1):69–75, 1998

O'Donnell BF, Faux SF, McCarley RW, et al: Increased rate of P300 latency prolongation with age in schizophrenia: electrophysiological evidence for a neurodegenerative process. Arch Gen Psychiatry 52:544–549, 1995

Robinson DJ, Merskey H, Blume WT, et al: Electroencephalography as an aid in the exclusion of Alzheimer's disease. Arch Neurol 51:280–284, 1994

Visser SL: EEG and evoked potentials in the diagnosis of dementia, in Senile Dementia of the Alzheimer Type. Edited by Traber J, Gispen WH. Berlin, Springer, 1985, pp 102–116

Zivin L, Marsan CA: Incidence and prognostic significance of "epileptiform" activity in the EEG of non-epileptic subjects. Brain 91:751–778, 1968

C H A P T E R   7

The Neuropsychological Evaluation

Select the single best response for each question.

7.1   A patient tells you that she has an IQ score at the 98th percentile. This corresponds to a *z* score of

A. −2.0.
B. +2.0.
C. +3.0.
D. +4.0.
E. 98.

The correct response is option B.

Neuropsychological tests rely on comparisons between a patient's present level of functioning and the known or estimated level of premorbid functioning. Very few people will obtain a perfect score, and most scores will cluster in a middle range. The plotting of scores as a distribution curve will most likely fall into a bell-shaped curve. Single scores are considered representative of a normal performance range, and for this reason many neuropsychologists tend to describe their findings in terms of ability levels rather than reporting scores.

Ability level classifications with associated *z* score ranges and percentiles follow:

- Very superior = >+2.0, 98–100
- Superior = +1.3 to +2.0, 91–97
- High average = +0.67 to +1.3, 75–90
- Average =−0.66 to +0.66, 26–74
- Low average =−0.67 to −1.3, 10–25
- Borderline =−1.3 to −2.0, 3–9
- Mentally retarded = <−2.0, 0–2 **(p. 224, Table 7–2)**

7.2   A test has validity when

A. It measures what it purports to measure.
B. It is given to the same individual at different times and the scores are consistent.
C. It was constructed with a large normative sample.
D. It is sensitive to brain damage.
E. It has high specificity.

The correct response is option A.

Tests have validity when they measure what they purport to measure. Most tests have small normative samples in the range of 30–200 individuals. Many neuropsychological tests offer a tradeoff between sensitivity and specificity. **(p. 225)**

7.3 Neuropsychological examinations include multiple measures of many cognitive functions. Multiple measures, which involve similar or related abilities, increase the _____ of findings.

  A. Specificity.
  B. Variability.
  C. Validity.
  D. Quality.
  E. Reliability.

The correct response is option E.

If a deviant score shows up on one test, other tests requiring similar skills are used to confirm the finding. Interpretations must also take into account the patient's education and occupational background, sex, and race to estimate premorbid functioning. **(p. 227)**

7.4 There is a tendency for left hemisphere lesions to produce a relatively depressed _____ in a neuropsychological test battery.

  A. Full-scale IQ.
  B. Performance IQ.
  C. Verbal IQ.
  D. Rey Complex Figure.
  E. Grooved Pegboard Test score.

The correct response is option C.

Left-hemisphere lesions tend to produce a relatively depressed Verbal IQ, whereas right-hemisphere lesions and diffuse damage produce a depressed Performance IQ. **(p. 228)**

7.5 The ability to hold information in mind while performing a mental task is called

  A. Processing speed.
  B. Visual acuity.
  C. Sensitivity.
  D. Working memory.
  E. Specificity.

The correct response is option D.

The ability to hold information in mind while performing a mental task is called *working memory*, and it requires attention and short-term memory. **(p. 229)**

7.6   The abilities involved in formulating goals, planning, effectively carrying out goal-directed plans, monitoring, and self-correcting are collectively called

A. Executive functions.
B. Motor functions.
C. Perception.
D. Praxis.
E. Constructional ability.

The correct response is option A.

Executive functions include abilities to formulate a goal, to plan, to carry out goal-directed plans effectively, and to monitor and self-correct spontaneously and reliably. Executive function tasks are difficult for patients with frontal lobe or diffuse brain injuries (Luria 1980). **(p. 233)**

7.7   The L, F, and K scales of the Minnesota Multiphasic Personality Inventory (MMPI) and MMPI-2 are also called the _____ scales.

A. Reliability.
B. Validity.
C. Neurological.
D. Compliant.
E. Symptom.

The correct response is option B.

The validity scales can provide information about the patient's cooperativeness and the likelihood that symptoms are exaggerated or minimized. **(p. 234)**

7.8   The most popular neuropsychological test battery in the United States is the

A. Category test.
B. Luria-Nebraska Neuropsychological Battery.
C. Halstead-Reitan Battery.
D. Dementia Rating Scale.
E. Mini-Mental State Exam.

The correct response is option C.

The Halstead-Reitan Battery was originally designed by Ward Halstead in 1947 to assess frontal lobe disorders. In 1969, Ralph Reitan added some tests and recommended it for all kinds of brain damage. **(p. 234)**

Reference

Luria AR: Higher Cortical Functions in Man, 2nd Edition. New York, Basic Books, 1980

C H A P T E R 8

Clinical Imaging in Neuropsychiatry

Select the single best response for each question.

8.1 The role of neuroimaging in neuropsychiatry has been evolving and in some areas remains controversial. In recent years, technical improvements have led to a broader use of neuroimaging. Which of the following would *not* be an indication for neuroimaging?

A. Cognitive decline verging on a diagnosis of dementia.
B. Traumatic brain injury.
C. Initial presentation of psychotic illness, regardless of age of patient.
D. New onset of nonpsychotic major depression in a 40-year-old patient.
E. Psychiatric symptoms in an alcohol-dependent patient.

The correct response is option D.

Neuroimaging is not indicated for the new onset of nonpsychotic major depression in a 40-year-old patient. Psychiatric conditions that *do* indicate a need for neuroimaging include psychiatric symptoms outside "clinical norms," dementia or cognitive decline, traumatic brain injury, new-onset mental illness after age 50, initial psychotic break, alcohol abuse, seizure disorders with psychiatric symptoms, movement disorders, autoimmune disorders, eating disorders, poison or toxin exposure, catatonia, and focal neurological signs. **(pp. 246–247, Table 8–2)**

8.2 The clinical benefit of neuroimaging can be increased by the judicious use of contrast agents. Which of the following statements about contrast-enhanced computed tomography (CT) is *not* true?

A. Contrast agents do not penetrate the intact blood-brain barrier (BBB).
B. Contrast agents may be visualized in the parenchyma of the brain in autoimmune disease, central nervous system infections, and tumors because of disruption of the BBB.
C. Vascular anomalies, such as arteriovenous malformations and aneurysms, can be visualized more readily by contrast-enhanced scans despite preservation of the BBB.
D. Xenon-enhanced CT (Xe/CT) may enhance identification of structural anomalies on CT, but cannot be repeated frequently and adds substantial expense.
E. Despite their greater expense, nonionic contrast agents are preferred because of their much lower risk of allergic reactions.

The correct response is option D.

Advantages of Xe/CT include lack of radiation or radiotracer exposure, good image resolution, and direct anatomical correlation. In addition, it is inexpensive and can be repeated frequently. **(pp. 247–252)**

8.3   The advent of magnetic resonance imaging (MRI) has significantly added to the anatomical detail that can be obtained by clinical neuroimaging. Although the procedure is safe for the vast majority of patients, there are some specific safety concerns that may limit its use. Which of the following is *not* true?

A. Cardiac pacemakers may be damaged by the magnetic field, which can alter programming and increase the risk of arrhythmias.
B. Pacemaker wires can develop dangerous levels of electrical current, leading to burns and/or movement of the wires and pacemaker.
C. Other implanted devices, such as cochlear implants, dental implants, and bone-growth stimulators, can be demagnetized or be moved by MRI.
D. Continuous physiological monitoring of a patient during an MRI procedure is not possible.
E. Caution is needed before subjecting a pregnant patient to an MRI.

The correct response is option D.

Although difficult, physiological monitoring of a patient during MRI is possible. Some manufacturers have developed MRI-compatible respirators and blood and heart rate monitors. If these devices are not available, the standard ones must be placed at least 8 feet from the magnet to avoid interferences. **(p. 263)**

8.4   The neuropsychiatrist must frequently choose among various structural neuroimaging protocols for patient evaluation. In this decision, the clinician should keep in mind that CT and MRI are each preferred for imaging of certain neuropsychiatric conditions. Which of the following conditions is better evaluated by MRI, as opposed to CT?

A. Acute cerebral hemorrhage with delirium.
B. Subcortical dementia from Parkinson's disease.
C. Calcified lesions from tuberous sclerosis.
D. Traumatic brain injury with physical evidence of skull fracture.
E. Acute psychosis without focal neurological signs when a "screening" examination is desired.

The correct response is option B.

All subcortical lesions (e.g., subcortical dementia from Parkinson's disease) are best evaluated by MRI. **(p. 264, Table 8–6)**

8.5   The caudate nucleus is the site of focal degeneration in Huntington's disease. The caudate nucleus, together with the putamen, receives projection inputs from numerous other areas of the brain and also has several outflow tracts. As such, this system can be regarded as having significant "relay" functions. Because of the complexity of these connections, many distinct neuropsychiatric symptoms may follow damage to the caudate nucleus. Which of the following is *not* a commonly reported deficit of caudate nucleus dysfunction?

A. Mania without episodes of depression.
B. Behavioral disinhibition.
C. Disorganization.
D. Aphasia.
E. Personality changes.

The correct response is option A.

The more commonly reported deficits of caudate nucleus dysfunction are disinhibition, disorganization, executive dysfunction, apathy, depression, memory loss, atypical aphasia, psychosis, personality changes, and predisposition for delirium. **(p. 269)**

8.6   The substantia nigra is composed of the pars reticulata and pars compacta. Which of the following is true regarding the substantia nigra and neuropsychiatric symptoms attributed to lesions of this area?

A. The pars reticulata has dopaminergic projections to the caudate nucleus and putamen.
B. The pars compacta sends efferents to the thalamus and subthalamus.
C. Lesions to the substantia nigra produce primarily cognitive, rather than behavioral, symptoms.
D. Mania is more common than depression with substantia nigra lesions.
E. Apraxia, ataxia, and aggressive behavior are common with substantia nigra lesions.

The correct response is option E.

Reported neuropsychiatric symptoms of lesions to the substantia nigra include primarily behavioral and emotional deficits (i.e., apraxia, ataxia, aggression, and depression), with less frequent reports of memory and cognitive deficits.

   The pars compacta sends dopaminergic projections to the caudate nucleus and putamen. The pars reticulata receives input from the striatum and sends efferents to the thalamus, subthalamus, and reticular formation. **(p. 279)**

8.7   The amygdala and thalamus have important anatomical connections and participate intimately in the regulation of emotion, behavior, and memory. Which of the following is true?

A. Lesions localized to the amygdala typically result in memory, rather than behavioral or emotional, symptoms.
B. Patients with amygdalar lesions will often present with diminished appetites for sexual behavior and feeding behavior.
C. Damage to the left medial thalamus produces deficits in visual memory.
D. Bilateral damage to the thalamus may result in either thalamic amnesia or dementia.
E. Disturbances in autonomic functions, mood, and circadian rhythm may be caused by lesions of the anterior, but not medial, thalamus.

The correct response is option D.

Bilateral damage is associated with severe memory impairment ("thalamic amnesia") as well as dementia.

   Neuropsychiatric symptoms of lesions to the amygdala are primarily behavioral and emotional. These include passivity or aggression; hypersexuality; hyperorality; hyperphagia; decreased fear, anxiety, or startle; and decreased link between emotion and memory. Damage to the left thalamus is associated with deficits in language and verbal memory. Damage to the right is associated with deficits in visuospatial and nonverbal intellect and visual memory. Damage to the anterior and medial thalamus can also result in disturbances of autonomic functions, mood, and the sleep/waking cycle (Bassetti et al. 1996; Lovblad et al. 1997). **(pp. 280–281)**

References

Bassetti C, Mathis J, Gugger M, et al: Hypersomnia following paramedian thalamic stroke: a report of 12 patients. Ann Neurol 39:471–480, 1996
Lovblad KO, Bassetti C, Mathis J, et al: MRI of paramedian thalamic stroke with sleep disturbance. Neuroradiology 39:693–698, 1997

C H A P T E R 9

Functional Neuroimaging in Psychiatry

Select the single best response for each question.

9.1 There are several different approaches to functional neuroimaging. Which of the following is *not* true?

A. Positron emission tomography (PET) and single photon emission computed tomography (SPECT) both use radioactivity to measure brain metabolism, cerebral blood flow, and neurotransmitter receptors, but PET is more widely available.

B. Functional magnetic resonance imaging (fMRI) employs levels of blood oxygenation to estimate neural activation.

C. Arterial spin tagging is used to estimate cerebral blood flow.

D. Magnetic resonance spectroscopy (MRS) assesses local chemical concentrations.

E. Magnetoencephalography (MEG) assesses magnetic fluctuations associated with regional brain activity.

The correct response is option A.

PET and SPECT both use radioactivity, but whereas PET has been difficult to find outside of academic research institutions, SPECT is available in most clinical centers. **(pp. 285–288)**

9.2 Regarding PET, which of the following is true?

A. The most commonly used radioisotopes in PET are oxygen 15 (^{15}O) water for imaging of metabolism and fluorine 18 (^{18}F) fluorodeoxyglucose (FDG) to image cerebral blood flow.

B. PET can be used to image neurotransmitters via a series of specific ligands.

C. PET resolution allows good visualization of small areas of cerebral activity.

D. The radiation exposure in PET with FDG is minimal so that a subject can be studied several times a year if needed.

E. PET with ^{15}O water has a long half-life, limiting the number of tasks participants can perform during scans.

The correct response is option B.

PET can be used to image neurotransmitters via a series of specific ligands.

The most commonly used radioisotopes in PET are ^{15}O water for cerebral blood flow studies and FDG to image metabolism. PET images lack the spatial resolution and anatomical detail needed to specifically identify smaller areas of brain activity. Because of radiation exposure, PET with FDG can only be used two to four times a year. Because of the short half-life of PET with ^{15}O water, 8–10 scans can be formed during a single imaging session. **(pp. 287–288, Table 9–1)**

9.3   Regarding SPECT, which of the following is true?

   A. SPECT has spatial resolution superior to that of PET.
   B. The radioligand [^{99m}Tc]hexamethylpropylene amine oxime (HMPAO) accumulates in endothelial cell membranes, but its activity remains constant for only 6 hours.
   C. Participants typically must receive radioligand injections in or near the scanning suite.
   D. SPECT is useful in diagnosis of dementia because it images neurodegeneration directly rather than inferring neural degeneration by decreased perfusion.
   E. Early SPECT studies using the cerebellum as a "control" region for cognitive processes must now be reinterpreted in light of the greater appreciation of the cognitive contribution of cerebellar function.

The correct response is option E.

Early SPECT studies in the 1980s and 1990s used the cerebellum as a "control" region because it was felt that the cerebellum had little to do with cognition. It is now apparent that the cerebellum is very actively involved in the cognitive process, hence the need to reinterpret the earlier studies.

   SPECT has spatial resolution inferior to that of PET. HMPAO is accumulated by endothelial cell membranes within several minutes, and it remains active for up to 24 hours. Because of this, patients can be injected away from the scanning room. SPECT may be beneficial in diagnosing dementing illnesses because areas of relative hypoperfusion, corresponding to neuronal degeneration, are visually apparent. **(pp. 288–290)**

9.4   Regarding fMRI and MRS, which of the following is true?

   A. The mechanism of relative oxygen excess versus metabolic demands at the heart of fMRI has been well-defined.
   B. Oxygenated hemoglobin is more paramagnetic than deoxygenated and thus "looks brighter" on T_2-weighted pulse sequences.
   C. The clinical availability of fMRI is limited by its not being available in a conventional MRI scanner.
   D. MRS has similar spatial resolution to fMRI.
   E. MRS has been used to elucidate brain loss in neurodegenerative conditions via use of N-acetyl aspartate (NAA).

The correct response is option E.

NAA is found in neurons and is absent in glial cell lines. Decreases in NAA reflect a diminished number of neurons and are proportionate to the brain loss in neurodegenerative disorders.

   The exact mechanism of relative oxygen versus metabolic demands remains to be determined. Oxygenated hemoglobin is less paramagnetic and looks brighter compared with deoxygenated hemoglobin on images created with T_2-weighted pulse sequences. fMRI is performed in standard, clinically available 1.5-T magnetic resonance scanners. MRS has limited spatial resolution. **(p. 290)**

9.5   Functional neuroimaging has been used to assess findings in mood disorders. Which of the following is *not* true?

   A. Based on many functional neuroimaging studies of mood disorder patients, a region including the medial prefrontal cortex, perigenual cortex, posterior cingulate cortex, amygdala, and extended amygdala is typically affected.
   B. The medial prefrontal cortex, perigenual cortex, posterior cingulate cortex, amygdala, and extended amygdala circuit is also often implicated in anxiety disorders.
   C. Unipolar depressed patients with pseudodementia have been shown to have decreased blood flow to the left medial prefrontal cortex and increased flow to the cerebellum.
   D. Depressed patients were shown to have increases in metabolism of the prefrontal and anterior cingulate cortices following treatment.
   E. In studies of serotonin type 2 (5-HT$_2$) receptor, depressed patients had lower specific binding on PET; this specific binding increased with antidepressant treatment.

The correct response is option E.

When examining with PET levels of 5-HT$_2$ receptor in depressed patients, researchers found that depressed patients had lower specific binding than that of control subjects and that treatment with antidepressants did not increase binding. **(pp. 301–303)**

9.6   The functional neuroimaging of schizophrenia is more developed than for most other neuropsychiatric illnesses. Which of the following is *not* true?

   A. There is a graded response between dopamine type 2 (D$_2$) receptor occupancy (as evidenced by PET) and clinical findings, in which clinical response, prolactinemia, and extrapyramidal side effects were found at increasing levels of receptor occupancy by a typical antipsychotic medication.
   B. A SPECT study of olanzapine, low versus high doses, found a dose-dependent degree of D$_2$ receptor occupancy but no significant differences in clinical measures.
   C. Cerebellar dysfunction in schizophrenia has been demonstrated by an fMRI study showing decreased cerebellar blood flow in schizophrenic patients.
   D. Schizophrenic patients with hallucinations and delusions have been shown to have increased metabolism in the left temporal, inferior parietal, and occipital temporal regions.
   E. Schizophrenic patients with increased levels of cognitive and behavioral disorganization have been shown to have increased blood flow in the anterior cingulate cortex and contiguous medial prefrontal cortex, left superior temporal lobe, and thalamus.

The correct response is option C.

Multiple recent studies indicate increased cerebellar blood flow in schizophrenic patients and lower than normal flow in bipolar patients when functional MRI is performed using an injected contrast. **(pp. 305–308)**

CHAPTER 10

Epidemiologic and Genetic Aspects of Neuropsychiatric Disorders

Select the single best response for each question.

10.1 Relative risk refers to the ratio of disease frequency in two different populations. The following five neuropsychiatric illnesses, all associated with cognitive impairment, have been found to have different relative risks when comparing morbid risk in first-degree relatives of affected patients to the rate of the illness in the general population. Which of these five illnesses has the lowest relative risk?

A. Schizophrenia.
B. Alzheimer's disease.
C. Parkinson's disease.
D. Huntington's disease.
E. Pick's disease.

The correct response is option B.

Alzheimer's disease has the lowest relative risk in first-degree relatives of affected patients.
(pp. 324–325, Table 10–2)

10.2 Which of the following types of study would be used by an investigator interested in identifying which chromosome is the site of a particular abnormal gene?

A. Molecular approaches.
B. Linkage analysis.
C. High-risk studies.
D. Segregation analysis.
E. Pedigree analysis.

The correct response is option B.

When trying to identify the inherited factors that contribute to the development of neuropsychiatric disease, the following questions and strategies have been developed:

- Is the disorder familial?—family studies
- Is it inherited?—twin studies, adoption studies
- What is being inherited in the disorder?—high-risk studies
- What "epigenetic" factors influence development of the disorder?—high-risk studies
- How is the disorder inherited?—segregation analysis, pedigree analysis
- Where is (are) the abnormal gene(s)?—linkage analysis
- What is (are) the abnormal gene(s)?—molecular approaches
- What is (are) its (their) molecular and pathologic effect(s)?—molecular approaches **(p. 324, Table 10–1)**

10.3 Regarding the genetic and epidemiological analysis of "complex disorders," all of the following are true *except*

A. Many neuropsychiatric disorders feature a complex pattern of inheritance.

B. The disorders exhibit incomplete penetrance, in which environmental factors may affect the degree to which a genetic disorder is phenotypically expressed.

C. The disorders exhibit variable expressivity, in which a single form of the disorder may have different phenotypic expressions.

D. Nonallelic heterogeneity refers to several genetic forms of a disorder following disruptions of a single gene.

E. Anticipation refers to the decreased age at onset and increased severity of clinical disease of a single illness over successive generations.

The correct response is option D.

Anticipation is a clinical phenomenon wherein the age at onset of disease decreases and the severity of disease increases in successive generations. Nonallelic heterogeneity refers to disruption in a number of different genes. **(p. 326)**

10.4 Huntington's disease is a well-delineated genetic neuropsychiatric illness. Which of the following is true?

A. The inheritance pattern is autosomal dominant with incomplete penetrance.

B. Juvenile-onset Huntington's disease or the "Westphal variant" features akinesia and rigidity instead of chorea and has a more benign course.

C. Common psychiatric symptoms include personality changes, dementia, psychosis, and depression; psychiatric symptoms may precede the onset of motor symptoms.

D. Anticipation, in which subsequent generations have an earlier onset of illness, is more likely with maternal, rather than paternal, inheritance.

E. Expanded CAG trinucleotide repeats on chromosome 4 are correlated with risk for disease and reliably predict age at onset of clinical symptoms in a given patient.

The correct response is option C.

Common psychiatric symptoms in Huntington's disease include change in personality, paranoia, psychosis, and depression. Affective disorders may precede other symptoms by 2–20 years.

The inheritance pattern of Huntington's disease is autosomal with complete penetrance. Juvenile-onset Huntington's disease has a more rapid and severe course of illness. Anticipation is more likely with paternal inheritance, and CAG repeat size is not particularly useful in predicting the age at onset. **(pp. 331–333)**

10.5 Parkinson's disease is another neuropsychiatric syndrome with significant epidemiologic and genetic considerations. Which of the following is true?

A. Parkinson's disease features loss of pigmented neurons in the zona reticularis of the substantia nigra.

B. Psychosis in Parkinson's disease is unrelated to advanced age or degree of cognitive decline.

C. Worldwide studies consistently find that Caucasians have a greater risk for Parkinson's disease than people of African descent.

D. Lewy bodies and Lewy neurites are pathological findings only in familial forms of Parkinson's disease.

E. The α-synuclein gene on chromosome 4 has been linked to Lewy body production in early-onset Parkinson's disease.

The correct response is option E.

The α-synuclein gene on chromosome 4 has been linked to Lewy body production in early-onset Parkinson's disease.

Parkinson's disease features loss of pigmented neurons in the zona compacta of the substantia nigra and in other brain regions. Psychosis increases in prevalence with advanced age and severity of cognitive impairment. Only in the United States do whites have higher prevalence and mortality than African Americans. Lewy bodies and Lewy neurites are present in nearly all forms of Parkinson's disease. (pp. 335–339)

10.6　Wilson's disease is a disorder of copper metabolism with dramatic neuropsychiatric symptoms. Which of the following is true?

A. Wilson's disease features the failure of a single pathway in copper metabolism.
B. Toxic amounts of copper accumulate in the liver and brain simultaneously.
C. Other than the brain and liver, tissues affected by copper deposition include the kidney and iris.
D. Siblings of affected patients, whose psychiatric symptoms include personality changes, depression, dementia, and psychosis, have a 25% risk of this disorder.
E. The inheritance pattern is autosomal dominant with incomplete penetrance, and preclinical screening tests can aid in prophylactic treatment.

The correct response is option D.

Siblings of patients with Wilson's disease have a 25% risk for developing the disorder.

In Wilson's disease, excessive copper is neither extracted by hepatocytes nor excreted into bile. Toxic amounts of copper accumulate first in the liver and then spill out into the serum to infiltrate the brain, kidney, and cornea. The basal ganglia are especially susceptible to the toxic effects of copper. Wilson's disease is an autosomal recessive disorder. (pp. 341–342)

10.7　Which of the following is true regarding Alzheimer's disease?

A. Cognitive impairment in Alzheimer's disease is more correlated with the presence of amyloid plaques, rather than tau-containing neurofibrillary tangles.
B. Cerebrospinal fluid (CSF) analysis in Alzheimer's disease includes high β-amyloid protein and tau protein levels.
C. Some epidemiological studies suggest both a protective effect of more education and an increased risk with lower levels of educational attainment.
D. The apolipoprotein-E (APOE) gene represents the "susceptibility gene" for Alzheimer's disease, and its effects are similar on all ages and populations studied.
E. In familial Alzheimer's disease, APOE ε4 homozygosity increases risk for illness but does not change age at onset.

The correct response is option C.

Some studies suggest that more education may be protective against Alzheimer's disease or at least delay the onset of obvious symptoms. Other studies have shown an association between lower level of education and Alzheimer's disease.

Cognitive impairment in Alzheimer's disease is more closely associated with the presence of tau-composed tangles and not the presence of amyloid plaques. CSF analysis in Alzheimer's disease includes low β-amyloid and high tau protein levels. The modifying effect of the APOE gene, the susceptibility gene for Alzheimer's disease, is likely age dependent and population specific. APOE ε4 increases the risk for Alzheimer's disease but decreases the age at onset of the disorder. (pp. 351–357)

10.8   Genetic linkage studies of bipolar disorder have identified several chromosomes with links to different variants of bipolar disorder. Which chromosome has been found in studies of the Old-Order Amish pedigree for bipolar disorder?

A. Chromosome 18.
B. Chromosome 21.
C. X chromosome.
D. Chromosome 11.
E. Chromosome 4.

The correct response is option D.

Although linkage studies in an Old-Order Amish pedigree initially provided evidence for a bipolar focus on chromosome 11, this was not replicated in other populations and an extension of the original Amish pedigree weakened the evidence. (pp. 370–371)

10.9   Regarding genetic and epidemiological aspects of obsessive-compulsive disorder (OCD), which of the following is true?

A. There is a 15% excess of males as opposed to females.
B. Females have a significantly younger age at onset.
C. Affected females with early-onset illness have a higher incidence of birth complications than males.
D. Early onset predicts a higher incidence of Tourette's syndrome and other tic disorders in relatives.
E. Linkage analysis and genetic mode of inheritance for OCD are clearly established.

The correct response is option D.

OCD co-occurs with tics and Tourette's disorder, especially in early-onset males. Early-onset OCD predicts Tourette's disorder and tics in relatives, suggesting a distinct risk group for OCD (Pauls et al. 1995).
   In a review of 11 studies, 51% of OCD patients were females. There is a significant difference of age at onset, with males having earlier onset (19.5 for males, 22 for females). Males with early-onset OCD have a higher incidence of birth complications than females. No linkage studies have been performed for OCD. (pp. 377–379)

10.10 Schizophrenia has also been subjected to numerous genetic linkage studies. Which chromosome has been established as implicated in the failure of the sensory gating phenomenon in schizophrenia, based on the P50 auditory-evoked potential?

A. Chromosome 15.
B. Chromosome 13.
C. Chromosome 8.
D. Chromosome 22.
E. Chromosome 6.

The correct response is option A.

The failure to inhibit the P50 auditory-evoked response to repeated stimuli has been linked to chromosome 15 in schizophrenia and other diseases such as Prader-Willi syndrome and Andersmann's agenesis of the corpus callosum, which can entail schizophrenia-like psychoses. **(p. 383)**

Reference

Pauls DL, Alsobrook JP, Goodman W, et al: A family study of obsessive-compulsive disorder. Am J Psychiatry 152:76–84, 1995

C H A P T E R   1 1

Neuropsychiatric Aspects of Pain Management

Select the single best response for each question.

11.1 Which of the following is true regarding cognitive and emotional factors in pain?

A. Patients report more pain during the workweek than on weekends (because novelty enhances pain perception).

B. Reduced pain perception during hypnosis involves inhibition of the anterior cingulate gyrus.

C. Whereas pain patients score higher on measures of depression, anxiety is not notably increased in pain states.

D. Severe pain in oncology patients is strongly associated with symptoms of major depression.

E. In the Dworkin et al. (1990) study, even a single pain complaint was associated with a substantially increased risk for major depression.

The correct response is option D.

Significant pain among cancer patients is more strongly associated with major depressive symptoms than is a prior life history of depression.

Novelty tends to enhance pain perception (e.g., pain is often reported to be greater during evenings and weekends, when people are not distracted by routine activities). Reduced pain perception through hypnotic analgesia is associated with activation of the anterior cingulated gyrus. Patients with pain score higher on measures of depression, anxiety, and other signs of mood disturbance than do those with little or no pain. It has been suggested that chronic pain amplifies or even produces depression. Depression is the most frequently reported psychiatric diagnosis among chronic pain patients. In the Dworkin et al. (1990) study, patients with two or more pain conditions were found to be at elevated risk for major depression, whereas patients with only one pain condition did not show such an elevated rate of mood disorder. **(pp. 420–421)**

11.2 Regarding the transduction of signals at peripheral sensory receptors, which of the following is true?

A. Mechanothermal receptors are the most common nociceptors.

B. Prostaglandins are known to directly excite pain fibers.

C. Polymodal C fiber receptors are likely responsible for transmission of "first pain" signals.

D. Cardiac muscle afferents can be stimulated by prostaglandins, histamine, and bradykinin.

E. Secondary hyperalgesia is primarily due to the actions of histamine, as serotonin does not affect peripheral nociceptors.

The correct response is option D.

Prostaglandins, histamine, bradykinin, and serotonin can stimulate cardiac muscle afferents.

Mechanothermal nociceptors activated by high-intensity heat or pressure are responsible for "first pain" signals. Prostaglandins alone do not excite pain fibers. Polymodal C fiber nociceptors, the most common of all nociceptors, are responsible for transmission of "second pain" signals. Secondary hyperalgesia is the result of increases in histamine and serotonin, which activate peripheral nociceptors. **(pp. 422–424)**

11.3   Regarding the spinal cord terminals of primary afferents and their projections, which of the following is true?

   A.   All somatic primary afferent cell bodies are in the dorsal root ganglia, adjacent to the spinal cord.
   B.   All primary afferent fibers terminate ipsilaterally in the dorsal gray matter.
   C.   Cells of lamina I are called marginal cells and are responsive to mechanical stimuli.
   D.   Lamina II is the nucleus proprius and is responsible for noxious stimuli, light touch, and pressure sense.
   E.   The spinothalamic tracts are composed of over 90% "crossed" fibers from laminae I, IV, V, VII, and VIII from the contralateral dorsal horn.

The correct response is option C.

Cell bodies in lamina I are termed *marginal cells* and are responsive to noxious mechanical stimuli.

All somatic primary afferent cell bodies, with the exception of the trigeminal ganglia, are in the dorsal root ganglia adjacent to the spinal cord. Most primary afferent fibers terminate in the ipsilateral dorsal gray matter, but a small number terminate in the dorsal gray matter of the contralateral side. Lamina II cells are known as the *substantia gelatinosa*. The nucleus proprius is made up of the neurons located in laminae III and IV. Axons from laminae I, II, V, VII, and VIII make up the spinothalamic tract, in which crossed fibers dominate, and 25% of all fibers ascend in the ipsilateral ventral quadrant. **(pp. 425–426)**

11.4   There are several opioid receptors with differential properties. Which of the following is *not* true regarding the μ opioid receptor?

   A.   Agonists to the μ receptor induce pain relief.
   B.   Agonists to the μ receptor decrease level of consciousness and may cause sedation.
   C.   Agonists to the μ receptor may induce respiratory depression.
   D.   Euphoric affect may follow μ receptor agonism.
   E.   Pentazocine is a prototypical agonist of the μ receptor.

The correct response is option E.

Pentazocine is a prototypical agonist to the κ receptor. A prototypical agonist to the μ receptor is morphine, which induces pain relief and causes sedation, respiratory depression, and euphoria. **(p. 433, Table 11–1)**

11.5 Regarding the use of antidepressants and other medications as pain adjuncts, which of the following is true?

    A. Among tricyclic antidepressants (TCAs), secondary amines are more effective at serotonin reuptake blockade, whereas tertiary amines are superior at norepinephrine reuptake blockade.

    B. Pain relief from antidepressants requires several weeks of dosing, as is true for relief of depression.

    C. Secondary amine antidepressants include nortriptyline, amitriptyline, and imipramine.

    D. Anticonvulsant drugs are likely to act by blocking voltage-dependent sodium channels in neurons and thus are indicated for neuropathic pain.

    E. Because of their generally more favorable side effect profile when compared with TCAs, selective serotonin reuptake inhibitors (SSRIs) now have a clearly established role in pain management.

The correct response is option D.

Anticonvulsants suppress neuronal firing and have been used to treat neuropathic pain because they block voltage-dependent sodium channels.

    Secondary amines block norepinephrine, whereas tertiary amines block serotonin reuptake. Pain relief following use of antidepressants is effective in only 2–7 days, as opposed to the 3–4 weeks needed for antidepressant effect. Secondary amines include nortriptyline, protriptyline, and desipramine. The role of SSRIs in pain management has not been proven equal to that of TCAs. **(pp. 435–437)**

11.6 Regarding the use of hypnosis in pain management, all of the following are true *except*

    A. Hypnosis works through two related mechanisms: peripheral muscle relaxation, and central perceptual alteration and cognitive distraction.

    B. Patients may be instructed to imagine that a painful body part is "numb."

    C. Patients may be told to imagine that painful tissue is "warm" or "cold" by using imagery.

    D. Research studies have demonstrated that hypnosis can result in a decreased need for pharmacological pain relief.

    E. Patients must be considered "highly hypnotizable" to have clinical relief from hypnosis for pain control.

The correct response is option E.

Two out of every three adults are at least somewhat hypnotizable. Highly hypnotizable individuals can use hypnosis as analgesia for surgery, but clinically effective hypnotic analgesia is not confined to those with high hypnotizability. **(pp. 445–446)**

11.7 The thalamus functions as a key "relay" center for the transmission of pain sensations. Which of the following is true?

    A. In the thalamus, spinothalamic neurons terminate primarily on the ventroposterolateral and submedius nuclei.

    B. The ventroposterolateral nucleus subserves the qualitative aspects of sensation.

    C. The centromedian nucleus is responsible for localization of impulses in space.

    D. Nucleus submedius functions are not clearly defined at this time.

    E. Projections from the ventroposterolateral nucleus to parietal lobe areas 1, 2, and 3 are central to the emotional aspects of pain sensation.

The correct response is option D.

The physiological functions and connections of the nucleus submedius are unknown.

In the thalamus, spinothalamic neurons terminate primarily on the ventroposterolateral and centromedian nuclei. The ventroposterolateral nucleus is involved with localization of the impulse rather than the qualitative aspects of sensation. The centromedian nucleus is involved in the qualitative aspects of nociception. Projections from the ventroposterolateral nucleus to parietal lobe areas 1, 2, and 3 have not been found to be involved with aversive or emotional aspects of pain sensation. **(p. 427)**

Reference

Dworkin SF, Von Koroff M, LeResche L: Multiple pains and psychiatric disturbance: an epidemiologic investigation. Arch Gen Psychiatry 47:239–244, 1990

C H A P T E R 1 2

Neuropsychiatric Aspects of Primary Headache Disorders

Select the single best response for each question.

12.1   Classification of headache according to the International Headache Society is important for clinical diagnosis and management. Which of the following symptoms would lead the clinician to rule out episodic tension-type headache?

   A. Nausea and vomiting.
   B. Pressing/tightening quality to the pain.
   C. Mild-moderate pain intensity; activities not prohibited by headache.
   D. Bilateral.
   E. Unaffected by routine physical activities.

The correct response is option A.

Absence of nausea and vomiting is specified in International Headache Society diagnostic criteria for episodic tension-type headache. **(p. 452, Table 12–2, Criterion D)**

12.2   Psychiatric comorbidity may be an important clinical consideration in the management of headache in patients. Which of the following is *not* true?

   A. A higher lifetime prevalence of major depression is seen in severe nonmigraine headache patients compared with headache-free patients.
   B. Depression is extremely common in patients with chronic migraine.
   C. Headache is a common physical complaint in depressed patients.
   D. Improvement in headache has not been shown to alter the patient's Minnesota Multiphasic Personality Inventory (MMPI) scores.
   E. Psychiatric comorbidity is associated with headache intractability.

The correct response is option D.

Improvement in headache has been shown to decrease MMPI scores.
   A higher lifetime prevalence of major depression is seen in patients with severe nonmigraine headache. Depression occurs in 80% of chronic migraine patients. Eighty-four percent of depressed patients experience headache. Psychiatric comorbidity is a predictor of headache intractability. **(pp. 454–455)**

12.3   The phenomenon of aura is an important consideration in many migraine patients. Which of the following is true regarding migraine aura?

A. Over 50% of migraine patients experience auras.
B. Aura is invariably followed by a headache.
C. Visual auras may consist of "positive" symptoms (e.g., flashes of light) and "negative" symptoms (e.g., scotomata or blind spots).
D. The fortification spectrum is an arc of scintillating lights that generally begins peripherally and then migrates centrally.
E. Auras of paresthesias are most commonly experienced over the hemiface and in the contralateral upper extremity.

The correct response is option C.

Approximately 20% of migraine patients experience auras, and headache follows aura only 80% of the time. The most common auras are visual, and they include both positive and negative symptoms. *Teichopsia*, or *fortification spectrum*, is an arc of scintillating light that often begins in central vision and then expands. Paresthesias are more common on one side of the face and in the ipsilateral hand or arm. **(pp. 458–460)**

12.4   Basilar migraine may present an ambiguous clinical picture. Which of the following statements is true?

A. Basilar migraine is seen only in persons younger than 30 years.
B. Basilar migraine is more common in males than in females.
C. Visual symptoms are characteristically bilateral at the onset of the aura.
D. Unlike classic migraine, many of the symptoms are bilateral.
E. Changes in cognitive status are unusual.

The correct response is option D.

Basilar migraine, once believed to be mainly a disorder of adolescent girls, has been identified in all age groups, although it is more common in women than in men. Visual symptoms usually involve loss of one-half of the visual field. Cognitive changes follow the visual aura quite frequently. Unlike classic migraine, many of the associated neurologic events are of a bilateral nature. **(p. 461)**

12.5   Regarding epidemiology and comorbidity of migraine, which of the following is true?

A. Migraine and major depression are each associated with an increased prevalence of the other.
B. The prevalence of migraine is greater for females than males throughout adult life, and this difference is greatest between ages 20 and 30 years.
C. Migraine is more common with higher intelligence.
D. Migraine increases the risk for epilepsy but not for stroke.
E. Personality instruments have consistently shown that increased neuroticism predicts the presence of migraine in subjects of both sexes; these studies have not been contaminated by other psychiatric pathology and were all well-controlled.

The correct response is option A.

There is increased prevalence of migraine in depressed patients and increased prevalence of depression in patients with migraine. Migraine is about three times more common in women than in men, and the gender ratio increases from menarche to age 42 years. No evidence has been found to connect migraine to socioeconomic status or intelligence. Migraine increases the risk of neurologic diseases (epilepsy and stroke) and psychiatric disorders (depression, anxiety, panic, mania). Many investigators have used the MMPI to investigate the personality of patients with migraine, but no control groups have been used, creating opportunities for selection bias. A statistically insignificant number of patients has shown increased neuroticism. **(pp. 463–469)**

12.6 Preventative treatment is often indicated for the migraine patient. Which of the following would *not* be considered a primary preventative treatment for migraine?

A. β-Adrenergic blockers.
B. Opioids.
C. Antidepressants.
D. Calcium-channel blockers.
E. Anticonvulsants.

The correct response is option B.

Opioids are not used in the prevention of migraines. The major medication groups used as primary preventive treatment for migraine are β-adrenergic blockers, antidepressants, calcium-channel antagonists, serotonin antagonists, and anticonvulsants. **(pp. 477–478)**

12.7 Cluster headache is a relatively rare but profoundly disabling condition. Which of the following is *not* a physical finding in cluster headache?

A. Severe unilateral orbital, supraorbital, and temporal pain.
B. Conjunctival injection.
C. Lacrimation.
D. Mydriasis.
E. Ptosis.

The correct response is option D.

Mydriasis (dilation of the pupil) is not present.
   Cluster headache frequency ranges from one attack every other day to eight attacks a day of severe unilateral orbital, supraorbital, and/or temporal pain that lasts 15–180 minutes. The headache is associated with conjunctival injection, lacrimation, nasal congestion, rhinorrhea, miosis (contraction of the pupil), ptosis (eyelid drop), or eyelid edema. **(p. 479, Table 12–13)**

12.8 Acute treatments for cluster headache include all of the following *except*

A. Oxygen.
B. Antipsychotics.
C. Sumatriptan.
D. Dihydroergotamine.
E. Lidocaine.

The correct response is option B.

Acute treatments of cluster headache include oxygen inhalation, sumatriptan, dihydroergotamine, and lidocaine. Preventive treatments include antipsychotics, corticosteroids, and indomethacin. **(p. 480)**

C H A P T E R   1 3

Neuropsychiatric Aspects of Disorders of Attention

Select the single best response for each question.

13.1   *Executive control* involves the operation of several neurobehavioral systems. When a subject is able to efficiently shift from one response alternative to another to meet environmental demands, this phenomenon is called

A. Intention.
B. Selection.
C. Initiation.
D. Inhibition.
E. Switching.

The correct response is option E.

Switching is the ability to efficiently shift from one response alternative to another in accordance with changing environmental demands. **(p. 493)**

13.2   The neuroanatomical basis for attention involves several specific structures. Which of the following is *not* considered a key structure in attention?

A. Reticular activating system (RAS).
B. Thalamus and striatum.
C. Dominant posterior parietal cortex.
D. Prefrontal cortex.
E. Limbic system.

The correct response is option C.

The key structures in attention are the RAS, the thalamus and striatum, the nondominant posterior parietal cortex, the prefrontal cortex, and the anterior cingulate gyrus and limbic system. **(p. 494)**

13.3   The dorsolateral prefrontal cortex circuit is important in maintaining response flexibility and "working memory." Lesions of this system may result in all of the following *except*

A. Perseveration.
B. Distractibility.
C. Cognitive slowing.
D. Cognitive disorganization.
E. Lability of affect.

The correct response is option E.

Lesions of the dorsolateral prefrontal cortex circuit result in perseveration, distractibility, impersistence, slowing of cognitive speed, impairment in abstraction and memory retrieval, cognitive disorganization, and flatness of affect. **(p. 495)**

13.4   The clinical assessment of attention may be assisted by the use of neuropsychological test instruments. Which of the following is a test of response selection and control or executive control?

   A. Wisconsin Card Sorting Test.
   B. Weschler Adult Intelligence Scale—Revised (WAIS-R): picture completion.
   C. Stroop Test.
   D. Paced Auditory Serial Addition Task.
   E. Continuous Performance Test.

The correct response is option A.

The Wisconsin Card Sorting Test is a test of response selection and executive control. Other neuropsychological measures of attentional domains include

- **Sensory selective attention**—double simultaneous stimulation, letter or symbol cancellation, line bisection, spatial cueing paradigms, dichotic listening, Wechsler Adult Intelligence Scale—Revised (WAIS-R): picture completion, orienting response, event-related potential (ERP) tasks
- **Response selection and control (executive control)**—motor impersistence task, go/no-go task, reciprocal motor programs, Trail Making Test, Wisconsin Card Sorting Test, Porteus Mazes Test, controlled word generation, design fluency, spontaneous verbal generation
- **Attentional capacity, focus**—Digit Span Forward, Digit Span Backward, Corsi Blocks, serial addition/subtraction, Consonant Trigrams, symbol-digit tasks, Stroop Test, reaction time paradigms, Paced Auditory Serial Addition Task (PASAT), Dichotic Listening Test
- **Sustained performance and vigilance**—Continuous Performance Test (CPT), motor continuation, cancellation tasks **(p. 499, Table 13–1)**

13.5   The assessment and classification of the level of consciousness are important to accomplish in an orderly and standardized fashion. If the patient exhibits spontaneous eye opening, eye opening in response to pain, roving eye movements, and/or blink in response to threat, but no awareness or meaningful responsiveness, this would be considered to be

   A. Locked-in syndrome.
   B. Akinetic mutism.
   C. Persistent vegetative state.
   D. Stupor.
   E. Confusional state.

The correct response is option C.

In a persistent vegetative state, patients may open their eyes spontaneously and in response to pain. They may have roving eye movements and may blink in response to threat.

Locked-in syndrome is characterized by consciousness and awareness but lack of verbal and motor responses. Akinetic mutism is characterized by amotivation, mutism, and minimal reaction to environmental stimuli. With stupor, the patient shows minimal cognitive or behavioral activity yet is arousable. In confusional state, the patient may be able to engage in conversation but exhibits slowness, incoherence, disorientation, and extreme distractibility. **(pp. 506–507)**

13.6   Hemineglect can be formulated as a unilateral attentional disorder. All of the following are true of the hemineglect syndrome *except*

    A. Patients fail to draw the left half of a drawing.
    B. Patients have measurable (though not complete) hemianopia on formal visual field testing.
    C. Patients may have hemisomatosensory neglect.
    D. Patients may deny "ownership" of the extremities in the neglected hemispace.
    E. Neglect affecting several sensory modalities supports the model of neglect as an attentional, rather than a perceptual, disorder.

The correct response is option B.

Patients with neglect syndrome as a result of a stroke have normal visual fields yet fail to look at certain spatial positions. **(pp. 507–508)**

13.7   Which of the following is true regarding attentional deficits and major depression?

    A. Depressed patients rarely complain of difficulty in focus and concentration.
    B. Focused attention and sustained attention are less likely to be reduced in depression than sensory selective attention.
    C. Attentional performance in depression remains static over time.
    D. Manic patients make errors typified by poor inhibition and errors of "commission," whereas depressed patients have low arousal and make errors of "omission."
    E. Depression rarely needs to be ruled out when evaluating other attentional disorders.

The correct response is option D.

Manic patients tend to make more errors of commission and fail to inhibit responding, whereas depressed patients make more errors of omission.

    Subjective complaints of problems with concentration and focus are among the symptoms that are considered in a diagnosis of depression. Sensory selective attention is usually less affected than focused and sustained attention. Attentional performance is often quite variable in depression. Attentional disturbance is the most common cognitive symptom associated with major affective disorders. Depression must be ruled out or factored in when assessing attention associated with other brain disorders. **(p. 512)**

13.8   Which is true regarding attention-deficit/hyperactivity disorder (ADHD)?

    A. Between 30% and 50% of child ADHD patients continue with disabling symptoms in adulthood.
    B. There may be wide cultural variance in the diagnosis of ADHD; for example, ADHD is diagnosed 10 times more often in North America than in Great Britain.
    C. Most ADHD patients have cognitive impairment on formal assessment.
    D. Poor performance on WAIS-R Digit Span, Arithmetic, and Digit Symbol subtests is pathognomonic for ADHD.
    E. Errors of both "omission" and "commission" are characteristic of ADHD subjects.

The correct response is option E.

Children with ADHD exhibit more errors of omission and commission than control subjects, and they also show more rapid deterioration of task performance over time. Between 11% and 31% of children with ADHD continue to be disabled in adulthood. ADHD is diagnosed nearly 50 times as often in North America as in Great Britain. Patients with ADHD have, for the most part, normal intelligence and do not exhibit major cognitive dysfunction. **(pp. 513–514)**

CHAPTER 14

Neuropsychiatric Aspects of Delirium

Select the single best response for each question.

14.1 Patients with delirium can present with a multiplicity of clinical appearances. Regarding the signs and symptoms of delirium, which of the following is true?

A. The majority of delirium patients manifest the "hyperactive" or agitated type.

B. The distinction between delirium and Lewy body dementia is often clear because of the rare presence of prominent psychotic symptoms in Lewy body dementia.

C. Delirium is more common in dementia due to Pick's disease and Lewy body dementia than in dementia due to Alzheimer's disease and vascular dementia.

D. Delirium in a patient with dementia has a substantially different presentation than delirium in a patient without dementia.

E. Diffuse electroencephalographic slowing is more than twice as common in delirium as in dementia and can thus assist the physician in differential diagnosis.

The correct response is option E.

Diffuse electroencephalographic slowing occurs in 81% of delirium patients versus 33% of dementia patients.

The majority of delirium patients have either mixed or hypoactive symptom profiles. The distinction between delirium and Lewy body dementia is difficult to make because the latter fluctuates in severity and involves prominent psychotic symptoms. The risk of delirium appears to be greater in Alzheimer's disease of late onset and in dementia of vascular origin compared with other dementias. Overall, the presentation of delirium does not seem to be greatly altered by the presence of dementia. **(pp. 526–527)**

14.2 Regarding the epidemiology and morbidity/mortality of delirium, all of the following are true *except*

A. Studies of the epidemiology of delirium have shown a 10-fold difference in incidence and prevalence rates in hospitalized patients.

B. More than 10% of elderly patients may be expected to be delirious on hospital admission, and nearly 50% are delirious at some point during hospitalization.

C. Hyperactive delirium has been consistently found to have a higher mortality rate than hypoactive or mixed types.

D. Excess mortality in delirium patients may be somewhat attributable to excessive age, dementia, or other systemic morbidity compared with nondelirious patients.

E. Increased rates on institutionalization and decreased independent community living have been frequently found following episodes of delirium.

The correct response is option C.

Hyperalert delirium patients have the lowest rate of mortality (10%) when compared with patients with hypoalert delirium (38%) or mixed cases (30%). **(pp. 529–531)**

14.3   The concept of delirium risk factors and precipitant events has important consequences for clinical management. Which of the following is true?

   A.   Medication exposure is a factor in less than 20% of cases of delirium.
   B.   Standardized protocols to assess cognition, sleep, sensory deprivation, and hydration status have been shown to reduce the number, but not duration, of delirium episodes.
   C.   Postoperative delirium is most common on the first postoperative day.
   D.   Low albumin level may predispose a patient to delirium, in part by increasing the bioavailability of medications.
   E.   Increased blood-brain barrier permeability predisposes to delirium, but this is of clinical importance only with central nervous system surgery, illness, or injury.

The correct response is option D.

Low serum albumin is an important risk factor for dementia. Hypoalbuminemia results in the greater bioavailability of many drugs.

   Medication exposure is implicated as a cause in 20%–40% of cases of delirium. Standardized protocols to address cognitive impairment, sleep deprivation, immobility, visual impairment, hearing impairment, and dehydration resulted in significant reductions in the number and duration of delirium episodes. Postoperative delirium occurs most frequently at day 3. Increased blood-brain barrier permeability is a risk factor for delirium, as occurs in uremia. A large multicenter study found age, duration of anesthesia, lower educational level, second operation, postoperative infection, and respiratory complications to be predictors of postoperative cognitive impairment. **(pp. 533–535)**

14.4   Anticholinergic activity (expressed in terms of atropine equivalents) is an important property in a medication's propensity to induce delirium. Among the following common medications, which one has the highest level of anticholinergic activity?

   A.   Prednisolone.
   B.   Cimetidine.
   C.   Ranitidine.
   D.   Theophylline.
   E.   Furosemide.

The correct response is option B.

Cimetidine has the highest level of anticholinergic activity. **(p. 535, Table 14–5)**

14.5   Formal cognitive assessment is crucial in the evaluation of delirium. Which of the following is true?

   A.   The Mini-Mental State Exam (MMSE) is useful to establish the presence of a cognitive disorder and reliably distinguishes delirium from dementia.
   B.   A weakness of the MMSE is its lack of items that directly assess frontal lobe and nondominant hemisphere functions.
   C.   The clock drawing test screens for cognitive disorders and distinguishes delirium from dementia.
   D.   The Confusion Assessment Method requires administration by a psychiatrist.

E. The Delirium Rating Scale—Revised–98 reliably distinguishes delirium from dementia and functions well with repeated measures.

The correct response is option B.

The MMSE has a limited breadth of items, particularly for prefrontal executive and right-hemisphere functions.

The MMSE is clinically important to document the presence of a cognitive disorder, although it is insufficient to distinguish delirium from dementia (Trzepacz et al. 1988). The clock drawing test is a useful screen for cognitive impairment in medically ill patients, but it does not discriminate between delirium and dementia. The Confusion Assessment Method is intended for use by nonpsychiatric clinicians in hospital settings. The Delirium Rating Scale—Revised–98 distinguishes delirium from dementia; however, because of some of its items, it does not function as well for frequent repeated measurements. **(pp. 536–538)**

14.6 The electroencephalogram (EEG) may be a helpful adjunctive test for delirium. The most characteristic delirium pattern on EEG is diffuse slowing. Which EEG pattern is seen with delirium tremens from alcohol withdrawal?

A. Low-voltage fast activity.
B. Diffuse slowing.
C. Spikes/polyspikes, frontocentral.
D. Left/bilateral slowing or delta bursts.
E. Epileptiform activity, frontotemporal or generalized.

The correct response is option A.

Delirium tremens is associated with low-voltage fast activity (Kennard et al. 1945). **(p. 539, Table 14–8)**

14.7 Delirium symptoms have been found to vary across different studies. In attempts to unify the clinical diagnosis of delirium, a Trzepacz (1999) study grouped symptoms into "core" and "associated" or "noncore" symptoms. Which of the following is considered an associated or noncore symptom?

A. Attentional deficits.
B. Memory impairment.
C. Perceptual disturbances.
D. Thought process abnormality.
E. Motoric alterations.

The correct response is option C.

Core symptoms include attentional deficits, memory impairment, disorientation, sleep-wake cycle disturbance, thought process abnormality, motoric alterations, and language disturbances. Associated or noncore symptoms include perceptual disturbances (illusions, hallucinations), delusions, and affective change. **(p. 541)**

14.8   Regarding psychopharmacological management of delirium, which of the following is true?

   A. Physostigmine is an attractive medication to reverse anticholinergic delirium and has a safe side-effect profile.
   B. Haloperidol must be used with caution in hemodynamically unstable patients on pressor support because it can reverse dopamine-induced increases in renal blood flow.
   C. Because of QT_c prolongation risk with haloperidol, it should not be used in patients with QT_c greater than 400 msec.
   D. As an alternative to haloperidol, intravenous droperidol can be used, although it can induce hypotension due to α-adrenergic agonism.
   E. Among atypical antipsychotics, clozapine is contraindicated in delirium because of its anticholinergic effects.

The correct response is option E.

Clozapine has significant anticholinergic side effects, and its use is contraindicated in delirium.
   Physostigmine reverses anticholinergic delirium (Stern 1983), but its side effects (seizures) and short half-life make it unsuitable for routine clinical treatment of delirium. Haloperidol does not antagonize dopamine-induced increases in renal blood flow (Armstrong et al. 1986). Haloperidol should not be used in patients with QT_c greater than 500 msec. Compared with haloperidol, droperidol is very hypotensive because of potent α-adrenergic antagonism. **(pp. 548–549)**

References

Armstrong DH, Dasts JF, Reilly TE, et al: Effect of haloperidol on dopamine-induced increase in renal blood flow. Drug Intelligence and Clinical Pharmacy 20:543–546, 1986
Kennard MA, Bueding E, Wortis WB: Some biochemical and electroencephalographic changes in delirium tremens. Quarterly Journal of Studies on Alcohol 6:4–14, 1945
Stern TA: Continuous infusion of physostigmine in anticholinergic delirium: a case report. J Clin Psychiatry 44:463–464, 1983
Trzepacz PT: Update on the neuropathogenesis of delirium. Dement Geriatr Cogn Disord 10:330–334, 1999
Trzepacz PT, Baker RW, Greenhouse J: A symptom rating scale for delirium. Psychiatry Res 23:89–97, 1988

CHAPTER 15

Neuropsychiatric Aspects of Aphasia and Related Disorders

Select the single best response for each question.

15.1   The clinical aphasias are classified according to functional deficits according to the model of Wernicke-Geschwind. Which of the following is true?

A. Writing comprehension is preserved in most aphasia syndromes.
B. Anomic aphasia can be usually differentiated from Wernicke's aphasia in that only the former has impaired naming of common objects.
C. Conduction and Wernicke's aphasia both feature fluent speech with notable paraphasic speech errors.
D. Transcortical motor aphasia and transcortical sensory aphasia can be reliably differentiated by the presence of normal speech fluency in the former.
E. Global aphasia, despite several functional speech defects, generally features preserved fluency.

The correct response is option C.

The principal aphasia syndromes vary quite a bit from each other when measured in six major language areas: 1) fluency, 2) auditory comprehension, 3) repetition, 4) confrontational naming, 5) reading (aloud and for comprehension), and 6) writing. However, both Wernicke's aphasia and conduction aphasia feature fluent speech with paraphasic speech errors. **(pp. 567–568, Table 15–1)**

15.2   For the examination of language function in the Wernicke-Geschwind model, which of the following is considered a major language area?

A. Word-list generation.
B. Repetition.
C. Automatic speech.
D. Prosody.
E. Speech mechanics.

The correct response is option B.

In the Wernicke-Geschwind model the six major language areas are fluency, auditory comprehension, confrontational naming, repetition, reading, and writing. **(p. 567)**

15.3 Broca's and Wernicke's aphasias are two of the aphasia syndromes best known to most psychiatrists. Which of the following is true?

A. Despite being caused by a left-sided cortical lesion, apraxia of the left upper extremity and buccal-lingual apraxia are common.
B. Prognosis for functional recovery may depend on the "depth" of the central nervous system lesion; cortical lesions are generally permanent, whereas internal capsule lesions tend to produce reversible aphasia.
C. Patients with Wernicke's aphasia generally experience a loss of normal speech prosody.
D. Because of the posterior superior temporal lobe of the left cortex location of the lesion in Wernicke's aphasia, a left inferior quadrantanopsia may be seen.
E. In the poststroke patient, the clinician may have to differentiate Wernicke's aphasia from delirium. The delirium patient will often exhibit speed with empty content, whereas the Wernicke's aphasia patient will be incoherent.

The correct response is option A.

Broca's aphasia is characterized by nonfluent verbal output and abnormal repetition, naming, and writing comprehension. Most patients have right-sided weakness, and apraxia of the left limb and buccal-lingual apraxia are common.

If the lesion is superficial and involves only the cortex, the prognosis for improvement is good. However, if the lesion involves the basal ganglia and internal capsule, the language defect tends to be permanent. The most striking abnormality of Wernicke's aphasia is a disturbance of comprehension; verbal output, on the other hand, is fluent, with normal word count and phrase length. Often a superior quadrantanopsia may be present. **(pp. 568–570)**

15.4 The syndromes of conduction aphasia and global aphasia may be encountered less often than Broca's and Wernicke's aphasias. Which of the following is true?

A. In conduction aphasia, repetition and naming are affected similarly.
B. In conduction aphasia, reading comprehension is invariably abnormal.
C. In conduction aphasia, when present, apraxia is limited to the right upper extremity.
D. Global aphasia refers to deficits in all language modalities and is often accompanied by a right hemiplegia, right hemisensory deficit, and right homonymous hemianopsia.
E. Because of the magnitude of deficits, global aphasia can only follow an infarction in the distribution of the middle cerebral artery from a single devastating stroke.

The correct response is option D.

Global aphasia is characterized by severe language impairment in all six areas and is often accompanied by right hemiparesis or hemiplegia, a right hemisensory deficit, and a right homonymous hemianopsia. It is usually caused by a complete infarction of the middle cerebral artery, although occasionally it is caused by multiple cerebral emboli to the left hemisphere.

Conduction aphasia features a prominent disturbance in repetition and sometimes abnormal reading comprehension; apraxia of both the right and left limbs is often present. **(p. 570)**

15.5   Which of the following is true regarding other aphasia syndromes and the analogous condition of aprosodia?

A. Transcortical motor aphasia is clinically similar to Broca's aphasia except that the patient retains the ability to repeat accurately.
B. Transcortical sensory aphasia features paraphasic errors but not echolalia.
C. Anomic aphasia is a specific syndrome with defined neuroanatomical location and is unrelated to other aphasia syndromes.
D. Patients with anomic aphasias rarely experience alexia and agraphia in addition to anomia.
E. The aprosodia patient's emotionless response more resembles a psychotic disorder than a mood disorder.

The correct response is option A.

Transcortical aphasia resembles Broca's aphasia in its decreased verbal fluency, but patients have near normal ability to repeat. It resembles Wernicke's aphasia in its fluent paraphasic output and decreased verbal fluency, but it differs in the tendency to exhibit echolalia. Anomic aphasia often follows improvement from other aphasias. Many patients also experience alexia and agraphia. No specific causative location has been found for it. Aprosodia is characterized by a flat, monotonous verbal output and decreased facial grimacing, which is often misinterpreted as depression. **(pp. 570–572)**

15.6   The psychiatric comorbidity of aphasia syndromes may have important clinical consequences. Which of the following is true?

A. The frustration of the Broca's aphasia patient in efforts at communication may lead to agitated gestures and expletives.
B. Depression is equally common in anterior- and posterior-hemisphere lesions that lead to aphasia.
C. Because of the frustration over communication failure and depression, suicide risk is particularly high in Broca's aphasia.
D. Posterior aphasia behavioral syndrome features mood disturbance but rarely psychosis.
E. Patients with posterior aphasia, despite other comprehension problems, usually can recognize their own recorded speech.

The correct response is option A.

Broca's aphasia patients may express their frustration at communication with agitated gestures and expletives.

Depression is more common and intense in patients with anterior aphasia. Some patients with posterior aphasia display impulsive behavior, which when combined with paranoia and unawareness, makes them potentially dangerous to others. Patients with posterior aphasia are often unaware of their language deficit and do not recognize their own recorded speech. **(p. 574)**

CHAPTER   1 6

Neuropsychiatric Aspects of Aggression and Impulse Control Disorders

Select the single best response for each question.

16.1   Regarding the epidemiology of violent behavior in the United States, which of the following is true?

A. Homicide is the leading cause of death of people ages 15–24 years.

B. Women are equally likely as men to die by homicide.

C. In cases of domestic violence, men are more likely to attack their domestic partner than are women.

D. In 50% of homicides, both perpetrator and victim are of the same race.

E. Nations with strict gun control laws have lower homicide rates than does the United States.

The correct response is option E.

Nations with strict gun control, such as England, Sweden, and Japan, have lower homicide rates than the United States.

In the United States, homicide is the second leading cause of death of people ages 15–24 years. Men are three times more likely to die by homicide than women. In domestic violence, women are more likely to attack their partner than are men. In 90% of homicides, both perpetrator and victim are of the same race. **(p. 580)**

16.2   Clinical assessment instruments may assist the clinician in evaluation and management of the violent patient. Which of the following is true?

A. Despite the development of more specific instruments, the Rorschach and Thematic Apperception tests remain definitive tests for evaluating aggressive behavior.

B. The Buss-Durkee Hostility Inventory requires clinician administration.

C. The Hostility and Direction of Hostility Questionnaire (HDHQ) is derived from components of the broader Millon Clinical Multiaxial Inventory.

D. The Brown-Goodwin Assessment (BGA) is clinician administered and includes clinical interview and review of available records.

E. The BGA contains 11 assessments, all of which address physical aggression against others.

The correct response is option D.

The BGA, based on clinical interview and/or review of medical records, has 11 assessments of both verbal and physical aggression.

Before more reliable instruments were developed, the Rorschach and Thematic Apperception tests were used to quantify aggression. Currently, the most widely used self-report assessment is the Buss-Durkee Hostility Inventory. The HDHQ, which is derived from the Minnesota Multiphasic Personality Inventory, contains five subscales, only one of which is relevant to aggressive behavior. **(pp. 580–581)**

16.3 Research has addressed the putative roles of various central nervous system structures in aggressive behavior. Which of the following statements is true?

A. Adults who have experienced physical abuse are much more likely to exhibit violent behavior as adults, a behavior that is directly related to the effects of head injury.

B. Destruction of the ventromedial nucleus of the hypothalamus in animal models leads to passive behavior.

C. Hamsters exhibit aggressive behavior after the administration of arginine vasopressin in the hypothalamus; this effect is blunted by the coadministration of a 5-hydroxytryptamine (serotonin) type 1B ($5\text{-}HT_{1B}$) receptor agonist.

D. In animal models, stimulation of the amygdala has a variable effect on aggression, depending on the animal's preexisting temperament.

E. Patients with temporal lobe epilepsy are more likely to demonstrate aggressive behavior in the ictal or immediate postictal period than in the interictal period.

The correct response is option D.

In animal models, stimulation of the amygdala has resulted in aggressive behavior that varies according to the animal's preexisting temperament. Research on the major brain structures involved in mediating aggression has focused on the hypothalamus, amygdala, and prefrontal cortex.

Many studies show an association between physical abuse and later aggressive behavior, although the connection between physical abuse, head injury, and aggression is uncertain. Destruction of the ventromedial nucleus of the hypothalamus in cats and rats produced aggression. Hamsters showed increased aggression following administration directly in the anterior hypothalamus of arginine vasopressin in conjunction with a $5\text{-}HT_{1B}$ receptor agonist. Patients with temporal lobe epilepsy may demonstrate hyperemotionality and increased aggression. Interictal aggression is much more common than ictal or postictal aggression. **(pp. 582–583)**

16.4 The prefrontal cortex has garnered a great deal of attention in the study of aggression. Which of the following is true?

A. As with temporal lobe epilepsy patients who behave violently, patients with frontal lobe injury and violent behavior typically show remorse for their violent acts after the fact.

B. Orbital lesions of the prefrontal cortex often result in impaired long-term planning and increased apathy.

C. Dorsal prefrontal lesions are associated with increased affective responses to stimuli encountered in the environment.

D. According to Soloff et al. (2000), patients with narcissistic personality disorder had a diminished response to serotonergic stimulation in prefrontal areas subserving behavioral regulation.

E. According to Raine et al. (1998), subjects who committed impulsive murders had impaired prefrontal cortex function when compared with predatory (nonimpulsive) murderers.

The correct response is option E.

The prefrontal cortex is associated with the social and judgmental aspects of aggression. Impulsive murderers have been shown to have impaired prefrontal function when compared with predatory murderers (Raine et al. 1998). Patients with prefrontal cortex lesions often express indifference, unlike patients with temporal lobe epilepsy, who show remorse for their violent acts. Orbital lesions of the prefrontal cortex are associated with increases in reflexive emotional responses to environmental stimuli (Luria 1980). Dorsal prefrontal lesions are associated with impairment in long-term planning and increased apathy. Borderline personality disorder patients have diminished response to serotonergic stimulation in areas of prefrontal cortex associated with impulsive behavior regulation (Soloff et al. 2000). **(p. 583)**

16.5   Much study of the neurochemistry of aggressive behavior has focused on the effects of serotonin. Which of the following is true?

A. Suicidal depressed patients have been found to have lower cerebrospinal fluid (CSF) 5-hydroxyindoleacetic acid (5-HIAA; a serotonin metabolite) levels than depressed patients without suicidality.

B. Among patients with Axis I disorders, CSF 5-HIAA levels are decreased in aggressive patients only if they also exhibit suicidal behavior.

C. The Linnoila et al. (1983) study cited demonstrated that decreased CSF 5-HIAA was decreased in all violent behavior, irrespective of premeditation.

D. Decreased brainstem levels in suicide victims have been reported in several studies, but this finding has been inconsistent across different studies.

E. Increased platelet transporter sites for serotonin, reflecting serotonin deficiency, are commonly seen in aggressive psychiatric patients.

The correct response is option A.

Suicidal depressed patients have lower CSF levels of 5-HIAA than nonsuicidal depressed patients; for example, Lidberg et al. (2000) found that murderers with a history of suicide attempts had lower CSF concentrations of 5-HIAA than other murderers.

Low CSF concentrations of 5-HIAA in aggressive patients, independent of their suicidal behavior, have been shown in patients with Axis I disorders by Stanley et al. (2000). Linnoila et al. (1983) reported reduced CSF 5-HIAA concentrations in impulsive violent offenders, compared with premeditated murderers. Decreased brainstem levels of serotonin and 5-HIAA are consistent postmortem findings in suicide victims. Decreased numbers of platelet serotonin transporter sites are found in aggressive conduct-disordered subjects and in aggressive institutionalized psychiatric subjects (Stoff et al. 1987). **(pp. 584–585)**

16.6   Which of the following is true regarding the neuropsychological and neuropsychiatric aspects of violent behavior and other clinical findings?

A. There is broad support for the finding that borderline personality disorder with violent behavior is solely a consequence of cognitive impairment.

B. Selective serotonin reuptake inhibitors (SSRIs) have been shown to decrease violent behavior but have not been shown to decrease nonviolent impulsive behavior (e.g., problematic gambling).

C. Paroxetine is the most thoroughly studied SSRI for impulsive behavior in borderline personality disorder.

D. High-dose fluoxetine in borderline personality disorder has been associated with decreased self-injurious behavior.

E. Tricyclic antidepressants have been consistently shown to be effective for aggression and impulsivity in borderline personality disorder, similar to their effects on depression.

The correct response is option D.

Markowitz (1990) reported that borderline personality disorder patients showed significant decreases in self-injurious behavior after treatment with fluoxetine 80 mg/day for 12 weeks.

There is limited support for cognitive impairment in patients with borderline personality disorder, although they are reported to be vulnerable to affective disruption and to be lacking in stable self-organizing strategies. SSRIs have been shown to decrease impulsive aggressive behavior, such as the severity of gambling in pathological gambling patients. Fluoxetine is the best-studied SSRI for the treatment of impulsivity and aggression. Tricyclic antidepressants have not been shown to be particularly helpful in decreasing aggression and impulsivity in borderline personality disorder. (pp. 589–591)

References

Lidberg L, Belfrage H, Bertilsson L, et al: Suicide attempts and impulse control disorder are related to low cerebrospinal fluid 5-HIAA in mentally disordered violent offenders. Acta Psychiatr Scand 101(5):395–402, 2000

Linnoila M, Virkkunen M, Scheinin M, et al: Low cerebrospinal fluid 5-hydroxyindoleacetic acid concentration differentiates impulsive from nonimpulsive violent behavior. Life Sci 33:2609–2614, 1983

Luria AR: Higher Cortical Functions in Man, 2nd Edition. New York, Basic Books, 1980

Markowitz PI: Fluoxetine treatment of self-injurious behavior in the mentally retarded (letter). J Clin Psychopharmacol 10:299–300, 1990

Raine A, Melroy JR, Bihrle S, et al: Reduced prefrontal and increased subcortical brain functioning assessed using positron emission tomography in predatory and affective murderers. Behav Sci Law 16(3):319–332, 1998

Soloff PH, Meltzer CC, Greer PJ, et al: A fenfluramine-activated FDG-PET study of borderline personality disorder. Biol Psychiatry 47(6):540–547, 2000

Stanley B, Molcho A, Stanley M, et al: Association of aggressive behavior with altered serotonergic function in patients who are not suicidal. Am J Psychiatry 157(4):609–614, 2000

Stoff DM, Pollack L, Vitello B, et al: Reduction of (3H)-imipramine binding sites on platelets of conduct disordered children. Neuropsychopharmacology 1:55–62, 1987

C H A P T E R 1 7

Neuropsychiatric Aspects of Memory and Amnesia

Select the single best response for each question.

17.1 Regarding conceptual classification of memory systems, which of the following memory functions is considered a component of working memory?

A. Central executive or "scratch pad."
B. Semantic.
C. Episodic.
D. Procedural.
E. Conditioning.

The correct response is option A.

Three aspects of memory have been identified: declarative, nondeclarative, and working memory. *Declarative memory* describes the conscious recollection of words, faces, things, and events. It is usually subdivided into *semantic* (which refers to the acquisition of factual information about the world) and *episodic* (which refers to the recording and recollecting of personal experiences). *Nondeclarative memory* is a classification for different tasks whose performance is not mediated by conscious recall. It is subdivided into procedural memory (applied to tasks that assess the acquisition of motor or cognitive skills), priming (the identification of objects from cues, as a consequence of prior exposure to the objects), and conditioning. *Working memory* provides a repository for briefly holding on to information, such as the name of a newly met person or a phone number. The central executive function is described as the organization for the retrieval or processing of information. **(p. 598)**

17.2 The acquisition of memory about the environment that is not cued to specific personal experiences and cannot be fixed as having been acquired at a discrete point in time is referred to as which type of memory?

A. Episodic.
B. Semantic.
C. Procedural.
D. Priming.
E. Conditioning.

The correct response is option B.

Semantic memories cannot be fixed as having been acquired at a discrete point in time. For instance, although most people know that Shakespeare is the author of *Hamlet*, few can recall when they first acquired this information. **(p. 598)**

17.3 Which of the following is true regarding specific memory functions?

A. Procedural memory refers to the acquisition of motor, but not cognitive, skills.

B. Procedural memory requires intact hippocampal function.

C. Physiological and environmental manipulations, such as cooling or central nervous system anoxia, disrupt short-term and long-term memory to an equal degree.

D. Electroconvulsive therapy (ECT)–induced amnesia's general transient nature supports the concept that memory retrieval, rather than storage, is affected by ECT.

E. Animal models with disruption in messenger ribonucleic acid (mRNA) synthesis decrease both short-term and long-term memory.

The correct response is option D.

ECT-induced amnesia is mostly transitory, which supports the theory that ECT affects the ability to retrieve memory, not its storage. *Procedural memory* refers to the acquisition of motor or cognitive skills, and several studies have suggested that it requires intact basal ganglia function. Cooling and anoxia can disrupt short-term but not long-term memory. Animal studies using agents designed to block mRNA synthesis have shown that long-term memory is selectively impaired and short-term memory is unaffected (Davis and Squire 1984). **(pp. 599–601)**

17.4 Although they are not invariably present in all patients with amnestic disorders, the four clinical characteristics of amnestic disorders include all of the following clinical symptoms *except*

A. Anterograde amnesia.

B. Retrograde amnesia.

C. Behavioral disinhibition or personality change.

D. Confabulation.

E. Relatively preserved intellectual function in other domains.

The correct response is option C.

The four typical characteristics of amnestic disorder include *anterograde amnesia* (the inability to acquire new information after onset), *retrograde amnesia* (the inability to retrieve information acquired before onset), *confabulation*, and *intact intellectual function*. **(p. 602)**

17.5 Which is true regarding Wernicke-Korsakoff syndrome?

A. The syndrome is caused by lesions of the temporal lobes, whereas the diencephalon is spared.

B. The acute phase, Wernicke's encephalopathy, classically features acute mental status changes, gait disturbances, oculomotor disturbances, and mononeuropathy.

C. The chronic phase, Korsakoff's psychosis, requires active hallucinations and/or delusions for diagnosis.

D. Dense anterograde amnesia and gradient retrograde amnesia are seen in the Korsakoff's stage of the illness.

E. Formal neuropsychological assessment generally reveals intact visuoperceptual and spatial organization functions, despite amnesia.

The correct response is option D.

Anterograde amnesia is dense, whereas recall of past events is poorest for events closest to the onset of the amnesia, but it improves for events in the more distant past (temporal gradient amnesia).

Wernicke-Korsakoff syndrome is attributed to lesions of mesial diencephalic brain structures and is normally seen in nutritionally depleted alcoholic patients. The acute phase (Wernicke's encephalopathy) features mental confusion, staggering gait, ocular symptoms, and polyneuropathy. The chronic phase (Korsakoff's psychosis) is characterized by anterograde and retrograde memory deficits. Neuropsychological tests usually reveal visuoperceptual and spatial organization deficits. **(p. 603)**

17.6   Depressed patients may present with memory complaints and/or findings of amnesia on clinical examination. Which of the following is true?

   A. Depressed patients with attention and concentration deficits may have impaired working memory as evidenced by the digit-span test.
   B. Despite complaints of memory dysfunction, depressed patients do not show defects in recall or recognition on formal testing.
   C. Depressed patients will generally complain of similar degrees of memory dysfunction on both "effortful" and "automatic" cognitive tasks.
   D. Depressed patients have greater difficulty with nondeclarative memory than with declarative memory.
   E. Depressed patients have greater access to pleasant than to unpleasant memories.

The correct response is option A.

There is mixed evidence that digit-span performance is impaired in major mood disorders (Breslow et al. 1980; Gass and Russell 1986; Whitehead 1973). It is usually thought that the deficits are a reflection of an attentional dysfunction with difficulty in concentration.

Depressed patients demonstrated deficits in recall but not in recognition (Calev and Erwin 1985). Depressed patients are more likely to manifest deficits in effortful than automatic cognitive tasks, and they have difficulties with declarative but not with nondeclarative memory. Depressed patients have greater access to memories whose affective valence is congruent with the current mood state (i.e., unpleasant rather than pleasant memories). **(p. 606)**

17.7   Regarding the syndrome of transient global amnesia (TGA), which of the following is true?

   A. Patients are usually elderly.
   B. The anterograde component of amnesia resolves before the retrograde component.
   C. During the amnestic period, disorientation (even to personal identity) is typical.
   D. Functional neuroimaging of TGA patients has shown transient decreased metabolic and functional activity in mesial temporal lobe structures.
   E. Cognitive functions other than memory are typically abnormal during an attack of TGA.

The correct response is option D.

Functional neuroimaging studies reported decreased activity in mesial temporal lobe structures during transient global amnesia.

In TGA, the patients, usually middle-aged, display retrograde amnesia and dense anterograde amnesia. The retrograde amnesia may resolve before the anterograde one. The amnesia is typically transient, lasting from minutes to several hours. During the amnesia, the individual is usually well oriented, with higher cognitive functions intact. **(p. 610)**

17.8 Amnesia following ECT treatments is a troubling side effect of this intervention. Which of the following is true?

  A. Differences in cognitive effects between bilateral and unilateral ECT treatments tend to be persistent, even well after the end of the ECT course of treatment.
  B. ECT typically degrades both declarative and procedural memory.
  C. There is a predictable, dose-response relationship between efficacy of ECT for mood disorders and the likelihood of postprocedural amnesia.
  D. Recent research suggests that patients most prone to post-ECT persistent retrograde amnesia are more likely to have had preexisting cognitive impairment.
  E. In post-ECT retrograde amnesia, memory for public events is less than for personal events.

The correct response is option D.

Recent research suggests that the patients most vulnerable to persistent retrograde amnesia are those with preexisting cognitive impairment and those who manifest the most prolonged disorientation after seizure induction (Sobin et al. 1995).

Differences in cognitive effects between unilateral and bilateral ECT treatment are difficult to detect a few months after the end of the treatment. ECT typically degrades declarative memory but not procedural memory. In post-ECT retrograde memory, information about public events is subject to greater loss than information about personal events. **(pp. 614–615)**

References

Breslow R, Kocsis J, Belkin B: Memory deficits in depression: evidence utilizing the Wechsler Memory Scale. Percept Mot Skills 51:541–542, 1980

Calev A, Erwin P: Recall and recognition in depressives: use of matched tasks. Br J Clin Psychol 24:127–128, 1985

Davis H, Squire L: Protein synthesis and memory. Psychol Bull 96:518–559, 1984

Gass C, Russell E: Differential impact of brain damage and depression on memory test performance. J Consult Clin Psychol 54:261–263, 1986

Sobin C, Sackeim HA, Prudic J, et al: Predictors of retrograde amnesia following ECT. Am J Psychiatry 152:995–1001, 1995

Whitehead A: Verbal learning and memory in elderly depressives. Br J Psychiatry 123:203–208, 1973

CHAPTER 18

Neuropsychiatric Aspects of Traumatic Brain Injury

Select the single best response for each question.

18.1 The pathophysiology of traumatic brain injury (TBI) has been examined from the perspectives of cellular metabolism and specific neuroanatomic vulnerability. Which of the following statements is true?

A. In TBI, damaged neurons have an acute metabolic need for increased blood flow, but the postinjury increase in blood flow is inadequate to meet these needs.

B. Secondary neurotoxicity includes calcium efflux, phospholipase activation, excitotoxin release, and lipid peroxidation.

C. One of the excitotoxic neurotransmitters in secondary neurotoxicity, glutamate, is increased in the cerebrospinal fluid (CSF) of TBI patients.

D. Hippocampal vulnerability to the effects of TBI is due to its predilection for damage by hypoxia and elevated intracranial pressure.

E. Functional alterations in hippocampal lesions correlate with decrements in memory and require cell death.

The correct response is option C.

Glutamate, one of the excitotoxic neurotransmitters in secondary neurotoxicity, is released during hypoxia and results in further neuronal damage (Becker et al. 1988; Faden et al. 1989).

After TBI, the damaged neurons have an increased demand for energy, but a decrease in cerebral blood flow occurs, resulting in a mismatch between needed and available energy supply. Secondary neurotoxicity is caused by calcium influx, phospholipase activation, inflammatory response, protease activation, excitotoxin release, and lipid peroxidation (DeKosky et al. 1998; Honig and Albers 1994). Hippocampal injury following TBI can occur even in the absence of hypoxia or elevated intracranial pressure. Functional alterations in hippocampal lesions may occur without neuronal cell death, and they correlate with decrements in memory. **(p. 627)**

18.2 The Glasgow Coma Scale (GCS) is a useful tool for clinical classification of neuropsychiatric functioning. Which of the following is true of assessment of TBI with the GCS?

A. Scores on the GCS range from 0 to 15.

B. Mild TBI is indicated by a GCS of 13–15 with loss of consciousness from 5 to 20 minutes.

C. Severe TBI requires a GCS of 8 or less, with abnormal findings on all three components of the scale.

D. *Decerebrate* posturing is considered a higher level of motor response than *decorticate* posturing.

E. The GCS is useful for both initial and follow-up assessment of level of neurologic function.

The correct response is option E.

The Glasgow Coma Scale (GCS) is a scale that ranges in points from 3 to 15; documents eye opening, verbal responsiveness, and motor response to stimuli; and may be used to measure the depth of coma, both initially and as a follow-up assessment. GCS scores for severe TBI are less than 10. Mild TBI is indicated by a GCS score of 13–15, a loss of consciousness of less than 15–20 minutes, and no prominent residual neurobehavioral deficits. Decerebrate (adduction, internal rotation of shoulder and pronation of the forearm) is a lower level of motor response than decorticate (abnormal flexion, adduction of the shoulder). **(pp. 628–629).**

18.3 Neuroimaging by various modalities is often important in the evaluation and management of TBI. Which of the following statements is *not* true?

A. Because the radiographic density of central nervous system (CNS) lesions may evolve, it is not uncommon for a computed tomography (CT) scan obtained 3 months after the head injury to reveal lesions initially unseen.
B. The frontal and temporal lobes are frequently the site of CNS lesions resulting in neuropsychiatric symptoms and are better visualized by magnetic resonance imaging (MRI) than CT.
C. MRI with morphometric analysis may demonstrate hippocampal atrophy and decreased thalamic volume in TBI.
D. MRI is preferred to CT for the imaging of contusions and subdural and epidural hematomas.
E. Single photon emission computed tomography (SPECT) should be used preferentially to CT and MRI where it is available.

The correct response is option E.

The American Academy of Neurology has concluded that there is insufficient evidence for the use of SPECT to diagnose TBI and that its use should be considered investigational (Therapeutics and Technology Assessment Subcommittee 1996). **(pp. 630–632)**

18.4 Regarding various neuropsychiatric clinical features associated with TBI, which of the following is true?

A. Anosmia, as manifest by deficiency in olfactory naming and recognition, may correlate with frontal and/or temporal lobe injury but is not of prognostic importance.
B. Substance abuse is associated with greater morbidity, but not mortality, from TBI.
C. Similar to the epidemiology of Alzheimer's disease, presence of the apolipoprotein-E (APOE) ε4 allele is associated with poorer functional recovery in TBI.
D. Personality changes following TBI are significant in a minority of patients.
E. TBI with damage to the orbitofrontal cortex results in a condition similar to the "negative/deficit" state of schizophrenia, with cognitive slowness, apathy, and perseveration.

The correct response is option C.

The presence of APOE ε4 predicts poor recovery in TBI, even after controlling for severity of injury (Teasdale et al. 1997).

   The presence of anosmia, which frequently occurs in patients with moderate or severe brain injury and is related to frontal and temporal lobe injury, is a predictor of major vocational problems. Substance abuse history is associated with greater morbidity and mortality rates in TBI. McKinlay et al. (1981) found that 49% of TBI patients had developed personality changes 3 months after the injury, and 74% had developed them after 5 years. TBI with orbitofrontal cortex damage results in behavioral excesses, such as impulsivity, disinhibition, hyperactivity, distractibility, and mood lability. Injury to the dorsolateral frontal cortex results in slowness, apathy, and perseveration, similar to the negative symptoms of schizophrenia. **(pp. 633–634)**

18.5   Mood disorders may follow TBI. Which of the following is true?

A. Patients with TBI do not differ significantly from noninjured patients with regard to their preinjury history of psychiatric illness.
B. The Beck Depression Inventory (BDI) is a reliable indicator of depression following TBI, even in the absence of formal psychiatric examination.
C. The increased suicide risk in TBI is primarily because of the incidence of major depression, with disinhibition from frontal lobe injury a minor factor.
D. The increased risk of depression after TBI has been shown to be approximately 25% at 1, 3, 6, and 12 months post-TBI.
E. The risk of depression after TBI is linearly related to duration of peri-injury loss of consciousness and duration of posttraumatic amnesia and is increased if there was skull fracture.

The correct response is option D.

In studies of patients who sustained acute TBI and were followed for a year, approximately 25% were shown to have depression when evaluated at 1, 3, 6, and 12 months after injury.

Several studies suggest that individuals who experience TBI have a higher than expected rate of preinjury psychiatric disorders. The BDI is not a reliable indicator of depression after TBI, because lability of mood and affect may be caused by temporal limbic and basal forebrain lesions. It is believed that the high incidence of suicide attempts in TBI is due to the combination of major depression with disinhibition secondary to frontal lobe injury. The incidence and severity of depression in TBI have not been found to be related to the duration of loss of consciousness (Bornstein et al. 1989; Levin and Grossman 1978), the duration of posttraumatic amnesia (Bornstein et al. 1988), or the presence or absence of skull fracture (Bornstein et al. 1988). **(pp. 636–637)**

18.6   Mild TBI has been associated with a constellation of neuropsychiatric symptoms called postconcussion syndrome. Which of the following is true?

A. Whereas the mechanism of injury is primarily diffuse axonal injury, neither structural (e.g., CT, MRI) nor functional (e.g., electroencephalogram, SPECT) assessments reveal abnormalities in mild TBI.
B. Whereas many postconcussion patients may complain of cognitive symptoms, these can infrequently be detected on formal neuropsychological examination at 3-month follow-up.
C. The majority of mild TBI patients recover cognitive function and experience decreased symptoms by 6 months.
D. Compensation for injury and ongoing litigation adversely affect recovery from mild TBI.
E. In the case of concurrent postconcussion symptoms and posttraumatic stress disorder (PTSD), PTSD symptoms typically spontaneously reverse earlier.

The correct response is option C.

The majority of individuals with mild TBI recover quickly and certainly at 6 months from the injury.
Structural brain imaging often does not reveal abnormalities in mild TBI, whereas functional imaging does. Most studies of cognitive function show deficits in memory, concentration, and speed of

information processing in mild TBI. Compensation and litigation do not appear to affect the course of recovery after mild TBI, and many patients return to work despite the continuation of psychiatric symptoms (Hugenholtz et al. 1988). Patients with mild TBI may develop PTSD, and although postconcussion symptoms decrease within 3 months, PTSD symptoms may not diminish until 3–6 months after the trauma. **(pp. 641–642)**

18.7 Psychopharmacological therapy may be invaluable in the management of symptoms following TBI. Which of the following is true?

A. Because of increased blood-brain barrier permeability and greater CSF penetration of psychotropic agents, both the starting and final doses of medications in TBI should be less than those for a neurologically intact adult.
B. Because of the likelihood of persistent risk for depressed mood in TBI, antidepressants generally should be continued indefinitely.
C. Because of the risk of additional amnestic symptoms, even with shorter courses of electroconvulsive therapy (ECT), ECT is discouraged in TBI patients.
D. Antidepressants are indicated for "pathological emotions" in TBI patients, even in the absence of a full-spectrum mood disorder.
E. Because they have been shown to dramatically increase the risk of seizures in TBI patients, psychostimulants are to be used only with great caution and with concurrent anticonvulsant therapy.

The correct response is option D.

Antidepressants may be used to treat the labile mood that frequently occurs with neurologic disease.
    Patients with brain injury are more sensitive to the side effects of medication. Consequently, doses of psychotropic medications must be raised and lowered in small increments, although patients may ultimately require the same doses used for patients without brain injury. Continuous reassessment is needed to determine whether continued use of medication is required. ECT can be used effectively after acute or severe TBI at the lowest possible energy levels needed to generate a seizure, increasing spacing of treatments. Overall, antidepressants may be associated with a greater frequency of seizures in patients with brain injury. Seizure control does not appear to worsen if psychotropic medication is introduced cautiously. **(pp. 645–650)**

18.8 Many medication classes are recommended for both acute and chronic management of persistently agitated/aggressive behavior in TBI. Which of the following medication classes is *not* recommended for the management of chronic agitation?

A. Benzodiazepines.
B. Atypical antipsychotics.
C. β-Blockers.
D. Buspirone.
E. Anticonvulsants.

The correct response is option A.

Benzodiazepines and antipsychotic drugs are indicated in the management of acute agitation and severe aggression but not in the management of chronic agitation. Atypical antipsychotics, anticonvulsants, serotonergic antidepressants, buspirone, and β-blockers are indicated in the management of chronic agitation. **(p. 654)**

References

Becker DP, Verity MA, Povlishock J, et al: Brain cellular injury and recovery: horizons for improving medical therapies in stroke and trauma. West J Med 148:670–684, 1988

Bornstein RA, Miller HB, van Schoor T: Emotional adjustment in compensated head injury patients. Neurosurgery 23:622–627, 1988

Bornstein RA, Miller HB, van Schoor JT: Neuropsychological deficit and emotional disturbance in head-injured patients. J Neurosurg 70:509–513, 1989

DeKosky ST, Kochanek PM, Clark RS, et al: Secondary injury after head trauma: subacute and long-term mechanisms. Semin Clin Neuropsychiatry 3:176–185, 1998

Faden AI, Demediuk P, Panter S, et al: The role of excitatory amino acids and NMDA receptors in traumatic brain injury. Science 244:798–800, 1989

Honig LS, Albers GW: Neuropharmacological treatment for acute brain injury, in Neuropsychiatry of Traumatic Brain Injury. Edited by Silver JM, Yudofsky SC, Hales RE. Washington, DC, American Psychiatric Press, 1994, pp 771–804

Hugenholtz H, Stuss DT, Stethem LL, et al: How long does it take to recover from a mild concussion? Neurosurgery 22:853–858, 1988

Levin HS, Grossman RG: Behavioral sequelae of closed head injury: a quantitative study. Arch Neurol 35:720–727, 1978

McKinlay WW, Brooks DN, Bond MR, et al: The short-term outcome of severe blunt head injury as reported by the relatives of the injured person. J Neurol Neurosurg Psychiatry 44:527–533, 1981

Teasdale GM, Nicoll JAR, Murray G, et al: Association of apolipoprotein E polymorphism with outcome after head injury. Lancet 350:1069–1071, 1997

Therapeutics and Technology Assessment Subcommittee of the American Academy of Neurology: Assessment of brain SPECT. Neurology 46:278–285, 1996

C H A P T E R   1 9

Neuropsychiatric Aspects of Seizure Disorders

Select the single best response for each question.

19.1   Which of the following is true regarding the International League Against Epilepsy (ILAE) classification scheme for seizure types?

A.   The anatomical locus for seizure syndromes (e.g., temporal lobe epilepsy) is preserved.

B.   The classification categorizes seizure syndromes, taking into account epidemiological variables such as age, sex, and concurrent illness.

C.   The main classification "branching" according to this scheme is partial versus focal seizures.

D.   Seizures that begin as partial seizures and then evolve to generalized tonic-clonic seizures are considered to then be "generalized."

E.   Absence seizures are considered focal because they do not have a notable motor component in most cases.

The correct response is option C.

The ILAE in 1981 revised the classification of epileptic seizures into partial versus generalized seizures. The anatomical classification of seizures no longer exists; the classification ignores attempts at explaining pathology and does not take into account age and sex. Seizures may begin as simple, progress to complex partial, and then secondarily generalize. Absence seizures are generalized, with loss of consciousness for a few seconds without any motor phase. **(p. 674)**

19.2   Which of the following is true regarding specific seizure syndromes?

A.   Complex partial seizures (CPSs) are experienced by a majority of seizure disorder patients.

B.   Absence seizures occur primarily in children and feature bilateral, synchronous electroencephalogram (EEG) spike waves between 6 and 7 Hz.

C.   When CPSs and absence seizures persist in status epilepticus, this represents a medical emergency, as is the case with tonic-clonic seizure status epilepticus.

D.   Temporal lobe epilepsy as a clinical syndrome is synonymous with CPSs.

E.   Temporal lobe seizures may be associated with 10–30 seconds of loss of consciousness accompanied by behavioral automatisms.

The correct response is option E.

Temporal lobe epilepsy may be manifested by brief loss of consciousness of 10–30 seconds, accompanied by chewing movements or "drop attacks."

CPSs are experienced by 40% of all patients with epilepsy. Absence seizures occur primarily in children, are generalized, and feature bilateral and synchronous spike waves of 3–4 Hz. With CPSs and absence seizures, consciousness is often preserved. These seizures do not necessarily constitute an emergency, unlike with tonic-clonic seizures, which are a true medical emergency. Temporal lobe epilepsy is not synonymous with CPSs because CPSs are restricted to patients who have local firing with defects of consciousness. (p. 675)

19.3   The clinical diagnosis of seizure disorder typically requires support from laboratory, neuroimaging, and EEG data. Which of the following is true regarding the findings in seizure disorder?

   A. The EEG is a definitive test, as over 90% of seizure disorder patients have abnormal EEGs, most often with "spike and wave" tracings.
   B. Increased serum prolactin, typically 3–4 times the patient's baseline level, is seen with equal frequency with generalized tonic-clonic seizures and partial complex seizures.
   C. Functional neuroimaging may be helpful, although single photon emission computed tomography (SPECT) is superior to positron emission tomography (PET) in the localization of interictal temporal lobe hypermetabolism.
   D. Clinical yield of EEG can be increased by placement of nasopharyngeal and sphenoidal electrodes, and both of these techniques equally increase the detection of seizure foci.
   E. A sleep EEG greatly increases the detection of focal abnormalities, such as a temporal lobe seizure focus.

The correct response is option E.

A sleep EEG increases the chances of picking up a focal abnormality, such as a temporal lobe focus, approximately fourfold. Approximately 20% of patients with epilepsy have normal EEGs, and 2% of patients without epilepsy have spike and wave formations. Increased serum prolactin is the major chemical diagnostic test for seizures; the increase is seen more often in major motor seizures and less frequently in partial complex seizures. PET is better than SPECT at detecting interictal temporal lobe hypermetabolism. Clinical yield of EEG can be increased with placement of sphenoidal electrodes. (pp. 677–678)

19.4   Nonepileptic seizures or "pseudoseizures" may complicate the clinical management of a patient with an apparent seizure disorder. Which of the following is true of pseudoseizure patients?

   A. The patients commonly also experience dissociative disorders rather than somatoform disorders.
   B. The seizures are often related to sleep.
   C. Motor symptoms have a characteristic abrupt onset and sudden remission.
   D. Neurological reflexes are preserved.
   E. Minor injury is common, as patients attempt to persuade the examiner of the legitimacy of seizures.

The correct response is option D.

With pseudoseizures, neurological reflexes are intact. Patients demonstrate somatoform disorders, particularly conversion, rather than dissociative disorders. Seizures are seldom sleep related, they often start and end gradually, and seldom result in injury. (p. 680)

19.5 The appearance of psychotic symptoms with seizure syndromes may render diagnosis and clinical management problematic. Which of the following is true regarding the differential diagnosis of psychotic symptoms in seizure disorders?

A. Some seizure patients experience periodic perceptual changes, alterations in level of consciousness, and intact memory for seizure events.
B. A chronic psychotic condition related to seizure disorder typically features complex hallucinations in several sensory modalities.
C. Seizure-related psychotic symptoms are generally communicated as being ego-syntonic.
D. Patients with atypical psychoses (i.e., psychotic conditions not clearly meeting criteria for schizophrenia) are more likely to have comorbid epilepsy than schizophrenic patients.
E. Among the atypical antipsychotic agents, clozapine is no more likely to lower the seizure threshold than other atypical agents.

The correct response is option D.

Patients with atypical psychosis seemed to have marked disturbance in their EEG, and the incidence of epilepsy was higher among them than among patients with schizophrenia or bipolar disorder (Mitsuda 1967). Some seizure patients experience periodic perceptual changes and have relative amnesia for seizure events. In chronic psychotic conditions, patients experience simple auditory hallucinations, paranoia, or other perceptual changes. Patients with seizure disorder and psychosis view their symptoms as ego-dystonic. It is well known that clozapine has a propensity to lower the seizure threshold. **(pp. 683–684)**

19.6 The differential diagnosis of seizure symptoms includes symptoms of various anxiety disorders. Which of the following is true?

A. There is a strong epidemiological association between seizure disorder and panic disorder, based on the presence of overlapping symptoms.
B. Dissociative symptoms are more characteristic of seizure disorders than of anxiety disorders, thus usually they can be used by the clinician to distinguish between the two illnesses.
C. A positive family history is much more likely in seizure disorder than in panic disorder.
D. Attacks of CPSs are usually shorter than panic attacks.
E. Anxiety due to seizure disorder will typically respond to antidepressants.

The correct response is option D.

Anxiety attacks in patients with CPSs are generally shorter than panic attacks.

There is a mild association between panic disorder and seizures (Neugebauer et al. 1993). Both seizure disorders and anxiety disorders present with dissociative symptoms: depersonalization, derealization, and déjà vu. In panic attacks there is a positive family history. Antidepressants may worsen the course of the illness in individuals with CPSs who develop anxiety. **(pp. 684–685)**

19.7 Comorbid mood disorders may complicate management of seizure disorders. Which of the following is true?

A. Patients with temporal lobe epilepsy have a modestly increased risk of suicidal behavior.
B. Neurosurgery for refractory temporal lobe seizures has been associated with a decreased recurrence of comorbid depression.
C. Seizures following the use of antidepressants is an idiosyncratic, rather than dose-related, phenomenon.
D. Treatment of depression in seizure patients rarely improves seizure control per se.
E. Selective serotonin reuptake inhibitors have been shown to be superior to other antidepressants for mood disorders in seizure patients and thus should be used preferentially.

The correct response is option B.

Forty-seven percent of patients with refractory temporal lobe seizures have shown no recurrence of depression following neurosurgery.

Temporal lobe epilepsy patients have a 25-fold increase in suicide risk. Most of the seizures following the use of antidepressants are dose related. In most cases, treating the depression often improves seizure control. To date, however, there is no evidence that any particular antidepressant is more effective than another. **(pp. 685–686)**

References

Mitsuda H: Clinical genetics in psychiatry. Bulletin of the Osaka Medical School Suppl 12:23–261, 1967
Neugebauer R, Weissman MM, Ouellette R, et al: Comorbidity of panic disorder and seizures: affinity or artifact? J Anxiety Disord 7:21–35, 1993

C H A P T E R   2 0

Neuropsychiatric Aspects of Sleep and Sleep Disorders

Select the single best response for each question.

20.1 Which of the following is true regarding sleep stages and their electroencephalogram (EEG) correlates?

  A. Sleep onset is determined when the alpha wave activity increases to greater than 50% of a given epoch (30 seconds of recording time).
  B. Stage II sleep features sleep spindles and/or K complexes, with delta-wave activity representing less than 20% of an epoch.
  C. Stage III sleep requires delta-wave activity for greater than 50% of an epoch.
  D. Stages I–IV are called non–rapid eye movement (NREM) sleep, whereas slow-wave sleep refers to Stage IV and REM.
  E. Young adults typically spend one-third of the night in REM sleep.

The correct response is option B.

Stage II sleep features sleep spindles or K complexes, with delta-wave activity occupying less than 20% of an epoch.

  The sleep-onset epoch is determined when the duration of alpha activity decreases below 50% of an epoch. Stage III sleep requires 20%–50% delta activity. Stages I–IV are collectively called NREM sleep, and stages III and IV are often combined and called slow-wave sleep. Young adults typically spend half of the night in REM sleep. **(pp. 698–699)**

20.2 *Sleep architecture* refers to the progression of sleep through various stages during a sleep period. Which of the following is true?

  A. Sleep onset in normal healthy subjects is into REM sleep.
  B. NREM and REM sleep alternate approximately every 180 minutes.
  C. Slow-wave sleep is predominant in the late part of a sleep period.
  D. REM sleep is predominant in the early part of a sleep cycle.
  E. Slow-wave sleep decreases with age and can even disappear with time.

The correct response is option E.

Slow-wave sleep declines after adolescence, disappearing completely in some elderly individuals.

  Sleep is entered through NREM sleep. NREM and REM sleep alternate approximately every 90 minutes. Slow-wave sleep predominates in the first third of the night. REM sleep predominates in the last third of the night. **(p. 700)**

20.3   Sleep complaints can be important features in many neuropsychiatric disorders. Which of the following is true?

   A. Approximately 20% of patients with a main complaint of insomnia have a psychiatric illness.
   B. Selective REM deprivation can be used to treat depression.
   C. Antidepressant medications increase REM sleep and suppress NREM sleep.
   D. Unlike other antidepressants, bupropion and trazodone suppress REM sleep.
   E. Patients with schizophrenia have excess rebound REM sleep following REM sleep deprivation.

The correct response is option B.

Selective REM sleep deprivation may alleviate depression. Thirty-five percent of patients with a main complaint of insomnia have a psychiatric illness (Coleman et al. 1982). Most antidepressant medication, with the exception of bupropion and nefazodone, suppress REM sleep. Patients with schizophrenia do not have REM sleep rebound in response to REM sleep deprivation. **(p. 703)**

20.4   Periodic limb movement disorder (PLMD) is a troubling condition for many patients. Which of the following is true?

   A. This condition was previously called nocturnal myoclonus.
   B. The upper extremities are more commonly affected than the lower extremities.
   C. Despite the limb movements, patients are not aroused out of sleep.
   D. PLMD occurs as a disturbance of paralysis during REM.
   E. Antidepressants are associated with decreased limb movements.

The correct response is option A.

PLMD was previously known as nocturnal myoclonus.
   PLMD affects the lower extremities, with associated brief arousals from sleep. It occurs primarily in NREM sleep, and it can occur in association with the use of antidepressants, renal disease, anemia, or folate deficiency. **(p. 707)**

20.5   Regarding pharmacological treatment of insomnia and related complaints, which of the following is true?

   A. Because of its high abuse potential, clonazepam is rarely prescribed for PLMD.
   B. Tricyclic antidepressants (TCAs) have little effect on slow-wave sleep, whereas selective serotonin reuptake inhibitors (SSRIs) increase it.
   C. Monoamine oxidase inhibitors (MAOIs) suppress both slow-wave sleep and REM sleep.
   D. Benzodiazepines have a more dramatic effect on slow-wave sleep than on REM sleep.
   E. The major advantage of newer-generation hypnotic agents (e.g., zolpidem) is the absence of memory impairment associated with their use.

The correct response is option C.

MAOIs are powerful REM-sleep suppressors and also diminish slow-wave sleep.
   Clonazepam is commonly used and is quite effective for PLMD. Most TCAs increase slow-wave sleep, whereas SSRIs generally decrease slow-wave activity. Benzodiazepines suppress slow-wave sleep and, to a lesser extent, REM sleep. Zolpidem has very rapid onset and is short acting; however, amnesia persists as a side effect. **(pp. 711–712)**

20.6 Which of the following is *not* a risk factor for the sleep apnea syndrome?

    A. Male sex.
    B. Middle age or older.
    C. Obesity.
    D. Micrognathia.
    E. Hyperthyroidism.

The correct response is option E.

Hyperthyroidism is not a risk factor for sleep apnea. Predisposing factors are being male, reaching middle age, obesity, micrognathia, and hypothyroidism. **(pp. 713–714)**

20.7 The parasomnias are a group of sleep behavior disorders that are conceptualized by overlapping of various sleep cycles. Which of the following is true?

    A. A patient with sleepwalking is generally easily awakened during an episode of sleepwalking.
    B. Patients with sleep terrors are usually troubled by vivid memories of the terror episode.
    C. Nightmares are more common in patients with schizotypal, schizoid, and borderline personality disorder.
    D. Bruxism is most common in stage III and stage IV sleep.
    E. REM sleep behavior can be distinguished from sleepwalking in that the REM sleep behavior patient is "aware" of the actual physical environment, whereas the sleepwalker is not.

The correct response is option C.

Individuals at risk for nightmares include those with schizotypal personality disorder, borderline personality disorder, schizoid personality disorder, and schizophrenia.

Sleepwalkers are difficult to awaken. Patients with sleep terror usually have amnesia for the episodes. Sleep bruxism can occur in any stage of sleep but appears to be most common during Stage II and REM sleep. A sleepwalker is usually aware of the actual physical environment, unlike a person with REM sleep behavior disorder. **(pp. 717–719)**

Reference

Coleman RM, Roffwarg HP, Kennedy SJ, et al: Sleep-wake disorders based on a polysomnographic diagnosis: a national cooperative study. JAMA 247:997–1003, 1982

C H A P T E R   2 1

Neuropsychiatric Aspects of Cerebrovascular Disorders

Select the single best response for each question.

21.1   Cerebrovascular disease leading to neuropsychiatric illness may arise from a number of pathophysiological mechanisms. Which of the following is true?

    A. Atherosclerotic thrombosis is approximately twice as common as cerebral embolism as a cause of stroke.

    B. Transient ischemic attacks are equally common with thrombosis and embolism.

    C. Cardiac sources of cerebral emboli commonly include arrhythmias, congenital heart disease, prosthetic valves, and myocardial infarction.

    D. Lacunae affecting the small penetrating cerebral arteries commonly produce mixed motor and sensory strokes.

    E. Intracerebral hemorrhage is accompanied by a severe, throbbing headache in nearly 90% of cases.

The correct response is option C.

Possible cardiac sources of cerebral emboli include arrhythmias, congenital heart disease, infectious processes, prosthetic valves, postsurgical complications, and myocardial infarction.

    Atherosclerotic thrombosis and cerebral embolism each account for approximately one-third of all incidents of stroke. Transient ischemic attacks almost always indicate that a thrombotic process is occurring, and only rarely is embolism present. Lacunae are the result of occlusion of small penetrating cerebral arteries and may be associated with pure motor or sensory deficits. Intracerebral hemorrhage is accompanied by a severe headache in only about 50% of cases. **(pp. 726–727)**

21.2   Cerebrovascular disease is associated with a series of systemic disturbances referred to as *multiple vascular risk factors*. Which of the following is *not* considered a risk factor for atherosclerotic thrombosis?

    A. Alcoholism.

    B. Hyperlipidemia.

    C. Diabetes mellitus.

    D. Hypertension.

    E. Cigarette smoking.

The correct response is option A.

Alcoholism is not a risk factor for atherosclerotic thrombosis. Risk factors include hyperlipidemia, diabetes mellitus, hypertension, and cigarette smoking. **(p. 726)**

21.3 Various neuropsychiatric syndromes have been described in association with cerebrovascular disease. Which of the following is true?

A. Major depression is associated with left frontal lobe and basal ganglia lesions, with strongest hemispheric correlation of risk occurring 6 months after cerebrovascular accident (CVA).

B. Minor depression, subsyndromal for major depression, is approximately three times more common than major depression after CVA.

C. Unlike depressive disorders, poststroke anxiety disorders are more common with right-sided CVA.

D. Poststroke apathy is more common as part of a poststroke depression (PSD) than as an isolated neuropsychiatric symptom.

E. Pathological laughter and/or crying poststroke have a similar prevalence to major depression.

The correct response is option E.

Both major depression and pathological laughing and crying have a 20% prevalence.

Major depression is associated with left frontal lobe and left basal ganglia lesions, with strongest correlation of risk during the acute period after stroke. Minor depression has a prevalence of 10%–40%, compared with 20% for major depression. Anxiety disorders are more common with left cortical lesions. Poststroke apathy is more common as an isolated neuropsychiatric symptom than with depression. **(p. 729, Table 21–2)**

21.4 PSD is the most thoroughly studied post-CVA neuropsychiatric illness. Which of the following is true regarding the phenomenology and clinical presentation of PSD?

A. Because of symptom overlap with physical causes of specific symptoms attributable to PSD, DSM-IV criteria must be modified for the accurate diagnosis of PSD.

B. According to a study by Lipsey et al. (1986; quoted in Robinson 1998), PSD and functional major depression patients had nearly identical symptom profiles.

C. Poststroke catastrophic reaction and hyperemotionalism are integral to the diagnosis of PSD.

D. According to PSD epidemiological studies, PSD is more common in community settings than in hospital settings.

E. PSD persists beyond 1 year in the majority of cases.

The correct response is option B.

Patients with major depression after acute stroke had symptom profiles similar to those of patients with functional major depression. It is not necessary to modify DSM-IV criteria for the diagnosis of poststroke depression because diagnosis with unmodified symptoms had a specificity of 98% and a sensitivity of 100%. Poststroke catastrophic reactions and hyperemotionalism are not integral to the diagnosis of PSD because they are also present in patients without depression. According to epidemiological studies, PSD is more common in acute and rehabilitation settings than in community settings (major depression, 22% vs. 13%; minor depression, 17% vs. 10%). Major depression after acute stroke has a duration of approximately 9–12 months, with the mean frequency of persistence of major depression beyond 1 year at 26%. **(pp. 731–732)**

21.5 Premorbid risk factors and comorbid physical and/or cognitive impairment may be important variables in the clinical management of PSD. Which of the following is true?

A. Cortical atrophy appears to be a greater risk factor for PSD than subcortical atrophy.

B. A family history of depression is more common in PSD patients with left-sided than right-sided CVA or nondepressed CVA patients.

C. Poor functional recovery leads to increased risk of PSD more than does PSD lead to poor functional recovery.

D. Patients with PSD are more likely than nondepressed CVA patients to exhibit post-CVA cognitive impairment; this relationship appears stronger for left-sided lesions.

E. PSD treatment studies have consistently shown improved cognition following successful antidepressant therapy.

The correct response is option D.

Patients with major depression and left-hemisphere lesions have greater cognitive impairments than nondepressed patients with comparable left-hemisphere lesions.

Subcortical atrophy appears to be a greater risk factor for PSD than cortical atrophy. Patients who developed major depression after a right-hemisphere lesion had a significantly higher frequency of family history of psychiatric disorders than did patients with left-hemisphere lesions. PSD leads to poor functional recovery because depressed patients may be hopeless about the future and less motivated to rehabilitate. Treatment studies of PSD have consistently failed to show an improvement in cognitive function, even when mood disorders responded to antidepressant therapy. **(pp. 737–739)**

21.6 Regarding randomized, placebo-controlled, double-blind treatment studies for PSD, which of the following is true?

A. Nortriptyline showed greater improvement than placebo for PSD without cognitive side effects requiring discontinuation of treatment in the active drug patients.

B. Trazodone was shown to improve Hamilton Rating Scale for Depression (Ham-D) scores in PSD more than did placebo.

C. The first SSRI with demonstrated efficacy for PSD was citalopram.

D. Fluoxetine was shown to be equally effective to nortriptyline for PSD.

E. Fluoxetine and nortriptyline were both associated with weight loss in PSD treatment.

The correct response is option C.

The first SSRI with demonstrated efficacy for PSD was citalopram.

Nortriptyline showed significantly greater improvement than placebo for PSD; however, some patients experienced significant side effects (such as delirium, confusion, agitation) that required discontinuation of the drug. Trazodone was shown to improve Barthel Activities of Daily Living scores more than did placebo. Nortriptyline has a significantly higher response rate than fluoxetine or placebo. Fluoxetine was associated with a loss of 8.5% of initial body weight, which was not seen in patients treated with nortriptyline. **(pp. 740–741)**

21.7   Which of the following antidepressants have been shown to be effective in the treatment of pathologic emotions after stroke?

A. Nortriptyline and fluoxetine.
B. Fluoxetine and citalopram.
C. Sertraline and nortriptyline.
D. Citalopram and nortriptyline.
E. Fluoxetine and paroxetine.

The correct response is option D.

Use of citalopram reduced the number of crying episodes by at least 50%, and use of nortriptyline showed significant improvements in Pathologic Laughter and Crying Scale (PLACS) score.
(pp. 747–748)

References

Lipsey JR, Spencer WC, Rabins PV, et al: Phenomenological comparison of functional and poststroke depression. Am J Psychiatry 143:527–529, 1986
Robinson RG: The Clinical Neuropsychiatry of Stroke. New York, Cambridge University Press, 1998

CHAPTER 22

Neuropsychiatric Aspects of Brain Tumors

Select the single best response for each question.

22.1 Which of the following is true regarding the epidemiology of central nervous system (CNS) tumors?

A. The incidence of metastatic brain tumors is twice that of primary brain tumors.
B. Among primary brain tumors, meningiomas are more common than gliomas.
C. The group of gliomas includes both astrocytomas and glioblastomas.
D. Over 90% of brain tumors are located supratentorially.
E. Pituitary adenomas are extremely rare, accounting for less than 2% of brain tumors.

The correct response is option C.

Gliomas include both astrocytomas and glioblastomas. **(pp. 753–754, Table 22–1)**

22.2 Demographic variables such as age and sex, as well as concurrent systemic and/or neuropsychiatric disease, may be critical factors in the presentation of CNS tumors. Which of the following is true?

A. In pediatric patients, medulloblastomas are the most common CNS tumor.
B. Gliomas are typically seen in elderly patients.
C. Despite the possibility of CNS tumors being heralded by neuropsychiatric symptoms, primary brain tumors are seen in only a small fraction of psychiatric patients.
D. The most common primary site for metastatic brain tumor is the gastrointestinal tract.
E. Because of their great expanse, the frontal lobes are the site of 40% of all CNS tumors.

The correct response is option C.

The prevalence of intracranial tumors in psychiatric patients, compiled from autopsy data from mental hospitals, is only about 3%.

The most common CNS tumors in pediatric patients are astrocytomas, whereas gliomas are more often seen in the middle-aged population. Secondary metastatic brain tumors come principally from lung and breast primary lesions. The most common location of an intracranial brain tumor is the posterior fossa. **(pp. 753–754)**

22.3 Whereas studies on this topic have lacked precision and controversy remains, specifics of neuropsychiatric symptom presentation may be of some clinical value in the evaluation of the suspected CNS tumor patient. Which of the following is true?

A. Tumors with rapid, aggressive growth are more likely to present with disruptive behavioral and cognitive states, whereas insidiously growing tumors are more likely to present personality changes or mood symptoms.
B. Meningiomas are much more likely to present with psychosis than other tumor histological types, irrespective of neuroanatomical location.
C. Generally, the three most important factors influencing neuropsychiatric symptoms from CNS tumors are tumor histology, neuroanatomical location, and associated neurological signs.
D. Because of the primarily anatomical cause of neuropsychiatric symptoms in CNS tumors, the patient's premorbid psychiatric history is of little relevance.
E. Unilateral CNS tumors are more likely to manifest neuropsychiatric symptoms than are bilateral or multifocal tumors.

The correct response is option A.

Rapidly growing tumors are more commonly associated with severe, acute psychiatric symptoms, such as agitation or psychosis, as well as with more obvious cognitive dysfunctions. Patients with slow-growing tumors are more likely to present with personality changes, apathy, or depression, often without associated cognitive changes (Lishman 1987).

No significant predominance of one tumor type over another was found in patients with psychosis secondary to brain tumors (Davison and Bagley 1969). The factors that most significantly influence symptom formation appear to be the extent of tumor involvement, the rapidity of its growth, and its propensity to cause increased intracranial pressure. Bilateral tumors and those with multifocal involvement appear to be more frequently associated with neuropsychiatric symptoms. **(pp. 756–757)**

22.4 Which of the following is true regarding tumors of the frontal lobes?

A. Tumors of the frontal convexities, called dorsolateral prefrontal syndrome, are associated with "pseudopsychopathic" symptoms, including irritability, lability, and poor social judgment.
B. Orbitofrontal syndrome features apathy, indifference, and psychomotor retardation.
C. Because frontal lobe tumors tend to remain localized, they rarely produce pressure effects and edema.
D. Mood symptoms, including both euphoria and depression, are frequent in frontal lobe tumors.
E. Psychotic symptoms in frontal lobe tumors typically include complex delusions and well-formed hallucinations, largely indistinguishable from symptoms of schizophrenia.

The correct response is option D.

Tumors of the frontal lobes are frequently associated with behavioral symptoms.

Patients with tumors of the frontal convexities present with apathy, indifference, and psychomotor retardation and have problems with sustained attention and/or sequencing. The orbitofrontal syndrome is characterized by changes in personality, irritability and lability, poor judgment, and lack of insight. Tumors of the frontal lobe may produce pressure effects and edema. Delusions secondary to intracranial tumors are less complex than those that occur in schizophrenic patients. **(pp. 759–760)**

22.5 Which of the following is true regarding tumors of the temporal lobes?

A. Psychotic symptoms in temporal lobe tumors include mood swings and visual, olfactory, and tactile hallucinations in addition to the more typical auditory hallucinations seen in schizophrenia.
B. Temporal lobe tumor patients typically experience affective blunting and social distancing similar to schizophrenic patients.
C. Neuropsychiatric symptoms caused by temporal lobe tumors can easily be differentiated from those of frontal lobe tumors.
D. Temporal lobe tumor patients exhibit personality traits indistinguishable from those of temporal lobe seizure disorder patients.
E. Whereas mood and psychotic symptoms are common in temporal lobe tumor patients, anxiety disorders are rare.

The correct response is option A.

Psychotic symptoms in temporal lobe tumor patients include episodic mood swings with suicidal ideation or attempts, and visual, olfactory, and tactile hallucinations, as well as the auditory hallucinations seen in schizophrenic patients (Tucker et al. 1986).

Temporal lobe tumor patients manifest broad-range and appropriate affect and interact with and relate to others in a relatively normal fashion. Neuropsychiatric symptoms associated with temporal lobe tumors tend to be similar to those seen in patients with frontal lobe tumors and may include depressed mood with apathy and irritability or euphoric, expansive mood with hypomania or mania. Anxiety symptoms appear to be quite commonly associated with temporal lobe tumors. **(p. 761)**

22.6 The clinician must know when to suspect a CNS tumor in a neuropsychiatric patient. All of the following signs or symptoms should lead to increased suspicion of CNS malignancy *except*

A. New onset seizures in an adult.
B. New onset headaches, with increasing frequency and severity.
C. Nausea and vomiting, particularly when associated with headaches.
D. Sensory changes.
E. Generalized neurological signs and symptoms, such as weakness.

The correct response is option E.

The neurological signs and symptoms should be focal, not generalized, such as localized weakness, localized sensory loss, paresthesias or dysesthesias, ataxia, and incoordination. **(p. 765)**

22.7 The psychopharmacological management of neuropsychiatric symptoms may be critical in relieving symptoms and restoring function. Which of the following is true regarding the specific considerations of psychopharmacological therapy of CNS tumor patients?

A. Because of the anatomic substrate of psychotic symptoms, full-dose antipsychotic therapy is usually needed.
B. Because they have been rigorously studied and found to be safe in this population, atypical antipsychotic agents are the treatment of choice for psychosis due to CNS tumors.
C. Antiparkinsonian agents potentiate the risk of delirium in brain tumor patients, particularly when combined with low-potency typical antipsychotic agents.
D. Because it lowers the seizure threshold in brain tumor patients, the use of methylphenidate is problematic in these patients.
E. Electroconvulsive therapy (ECT) remains contraindicated in brain tumor patients with mood symptoms.

The correct response is option C.

Antiparkinsonian agents have a greater likelihood of causing or contributing to delirium, especially when combined with low-potency neuroleptics.

In patients with "organic" psychotic disorders, the therapeutically effective dose of an antipsychotic is often lower than that required for the treatment of primary "functional" psychoses. Few studies have been conducted on the efficacy of the newer atypical antipsychotics in the treatment of psychotic symptoms in brain tumor patients. Methylphenidate has been shown to be effective as an antidepressant in brain tumor patients because it is well tolerated and does not lower the seizure threshold. When pharmacologic treatments have failed, ECT should be given serious consideration. (pp. 774–775)

References

Davison K, Bagley CR: Schizophrenia-like psychoses associated with organic disorders of the central nervous system: a review of the literature, in Current Problems in Neuropsychiatry: Schizophrenia, Epilepsy, the Temporal Lobe (British Journal of Psychiatry Special Publication No 4). Edited by Harrington RN. London, UK, Headley Brothers, 1969, pp 126–130

Lishman WA: Organic Psychiatry: The Psychological Consequences of Cerebral Disorder. New York, Oxford University Press, 1987

Tucker GJ, Price TRP, Johnson VB, et al: Phenomenology of temporal lobe dysfunction: a link to atypical psychosis: a series of cases. J Nerv Ment Dis 174:348–356, 1986

C H A P T E R   2 3

Neuropsychiatric Aspects of Human Immunodeficiency Virus Infection of the Central Nervous System

Select the single best response for each question.

23.1   Neuropsychiatric illnesses resulting from human immunodeficiency virus (HIV) disease are of major importance to all clinicians working with these patients. Which of the following is true?

   A. The most common neuropsychiatric illness in HIV disease is psychotic disorder.
   B. Cognitive impairment may present early in the course of HIV disease but is largely unrelated to disease progression.
   C. Neuropathological examination of the brains of HIV-infected patients characteristically reveals more dramatic widened sulcal spaces, as opposed to ventricular atrophy.
   D. Because HIV dementia is considered a subcortical dementia, histological study of the cortex reveals minimal loss of dendritic area.
   E. HIV has been detected in the central nervous system (CNS) within 14 days of infection, supporting a primary role for HIV in neuropsychiatric illness.

The correct response is option E.

Direct brain infection by HIV is now widely believed to be the likely cause of related cognitive and other neurobehavioral disorders (Janssen et al. 1991). HIV-1 has been found in the CNS 14 days after the initial infection.

   The most common CNS complication is cognitive impairment of sufficient severity to warrant the diagnosis of dementia. The prevalence and severity of cognitive impairment increases as the diseases progresses (Heaton et al. 1995). Gross examination of the brain reveals that the white matter, subcortical structures, and vacuolar myelopathy of the spinal cord are commonly involved. In addition, extensive ventricular atrophy is found. Wiley et al. (1991) found up to a 40% loss of cortical dendritic area. **(pp. 784–785)**

23.2   Which of the following pairs are the most common opportunistic CNS infections in HIV?

   A. *Toxoplasma gondii* and *Candida albicans.*
   B. *Cryptococcus neoformans* and *Candida albicans.*
   C. *Aspergillus fumigatus* and *Toxoplasma gondii.*
   D. *Cryptococcus neoformans* and *Toxoplasma gondii.*
   E. *Candida albicans* and *Aspergillus fumigatus.*

The correct response is option D.

Toxoplasma gondii is the most common opportunistic infection in acquired immunodeficiency syndrome (AIDS) and may present as a focal or diffuse cognitive or affective disturbance. *Cryptococcus neoformans*, the other common AIDS-related intracranial infection, presents principally as a meningitis, with headache (Lipton 1991), altered mental status, nuchal rigidity, fever, and nausea and vomiting. **(p. 787)**

23.3   Cerebrospinal fluid (CSF) studies must be considered in evaluation of mental status changes in patients with HIV disease. Which of the following is true?

A. The amount of CSF virus and antibodies correlate directly with degree of cognitive impairment.
B. CSF β_2-microglobulin is a sensitive marker for dementia severity.
C. CSF homovanillic acid (HVA) is decreased in HIV and directly correlates with severity of dementia.
D. Whereas depressive and anxiety symptoms are common in HIV patients, they have not yet been correlated to CSF immune function markers.
E. Increased levels of quinolinic acid are seen in HIV dementia but not in CNS opportunistic infections in the absence of HIV dementia.

The correct response is option B.

The concentration of CSF β_2-microglobulin is highly correlated with both dementia severity and level of systemic disease.

   The amount of CSF virus and antibody has been found to be correlated with severity of neurological or cognitive symptomatology (Reboul et al. 1989). CSF levels of HVA were lower in HIV patients, and no direct relation was found between HVA levels and severity of dementia. A relationship between depressive and anxiety symptoms and CSF immune function markers has been found in HIV-positive patients (Praus et al. 1990). The level of quinolinic acid is related to severity of dementia/clinical status (Heyes et al. 1991). In patients with early-stage disease, quinolinic acid levels were twice those of non-HIV-infected subjects, and more than 20 times normal levels were detected in patients with severe dementia or CNS AIDS involvement. **(pp. 790–791)**

23.4   The specific neurobehavioral assessment of HIV dementia may help classification of HIV-related cognitive symptoms. Which of the following is true?

A. Symptoms of deficient memory registration, storage, and retrieval and decreased psychomotor speed and motor function are considered cortical symptoms.
B. Symptoms such as aphasia, agnosia, and apraxia are generally present early in the disease process.
C. Vague cognitive symptoms of decreased "cognitive efficiency" are seen often in at least 20% of HIV patients during the initial stages of the disease.
D. Severe HIV dementia is infrequently associated with psychotic symptoms.
E. Classical frontal-lobe symptoms, such as conceptualization and problem-solving difficulties, are restricted to the late stages of HIV dementia.

The correct response is option C.

Subclinical cognitive inefficiencies occur in more than 20% of asymptomatic HIV-1 infected individuals.

Symptoms of deficient memory registration, storage, retrieval, and decreased psychomotor speed or fine motor function are considered subcortical symptoms. Aphasia, agnosia, apraxia, and other sensory-perceptual functions can be present in AIDS but usually not until later in the course of the disease, perhaps as a result of some focal opportunistic infection. Psychotic symptoms, such as severe hallucinations and delusions, are one of the late signs of HIV-related neurobehavioral impairment, whereas conceptualization difficulties and problem-solving difficulties are an early sign. **(pp. 792–794)**

23.5   Psychopharmacological interventions are of great importance in HIV disease but are subject to several considerations. Which of the following is true?

   A. Because of the nature of the CNS neuropathology, HIV patients with delirium typically require higher doses of antipsychotic agents than do other delirium patients.
   B. Management of depression is especially crucial because HIV-affected patients have a suicide risk twice that of the general population.
   C. Psychostimulant therapy for depression has been demonstrated to be similarly effective to antidepressants for HIV-associated depression.
   D. Among antidepressants for HIV-associated depression, citalopram, nefazodone, venlafaxine, and mirtazapine are the weakest P450 3A4 inhibitors.
   E. β-Blockers are generally safe for chronic use for anxiety disorders in HIV disease because they do not produce dependence.

The correct response is option C.

In HIV-infected patients, treatment with the psychostimulant methylphenidate was associated with a remission of depressive symptoms that was statistically indistinguishable from that achieved with the tricyclic antidepressant desipramine (Fernandez et al. 1995).

HIV-positive patients are often more sensitive to neuroleptics and may require lower doses than do other delirium patients (Fernandez et al. 1989). The relative risk of suicide in AIDS patients was found to be 66.2 times that of the general population (Marzuk et al. 1988). Citalopram, nefazodone venlafaxine, and mirtazapine are the weakest 2D6 isoenzyme inhibitors (Greenblatt et al. 1998). β-Blockers are generally not used for the treatment of anxiety in AIDS patients because of their propensity to result in hypotensive episodes. **(pp. 797–801)**

References

Fernandez F, Levy JK, Mansell PWA: Management of delirium in terminally ill AIDS patients. Int J Psychiatry Med 19:165–172, 1989

Fernandez F, Levy JK, Sampley HR, et al: Effects of methylphenidate in HIV-related depression: a comparative trial with desipramine. Int J Psychiatry Med 25:53–67, 1995

Greenblatt DJ, VonMolke LL, Harmatz JS, et al: Drug interactions with newer antidepressants: role of human cytochromes P450. J Clin Psychiatry 59 (suppl 15):19–27, 1998

Heaton RK, Grant I, Butters N, et al: The HNRC 500—neuropsychology of HIV infection at different disease stages. Journal of the International Neuropsychological Society 1:231–251, 1995

Heyes MP, Brew BJ, Martin A, et al: Quinolinic acid in cerebrospinal fluid and serum in HIV-1 infection: relationship to clinical neurological status. Ann Neurol 29:202–209, 1991

Janssen RS, Cornblath DR, Epstein LG, and the Working Group of the American Academy of Neurology AIDS Task Force: Nomenclature and research case definitions for neurologic manifestations of human immunodeficiency virus-type 1 (HIV-1) infection. Neurology 41:778–785, 1991

Lipton SA: Calcium channel antagonists and human immunodeficiency virus coat protein-mediated neuronal injury. Ann Neurol 30:110–114, 1991

Marzuk PM, Tierney H, Tardiff K, et al: Increased risk of suicide in persons with AIDS. JAMA 259:1333–1337, 1988

Praus DJ, Brown GR, Rundell JR, et al: Associations between cerebrospinal fluid parameters and high degrees of anxiety or depression in United States Air Force personnel infected with human immunodeficiency virus. J Nerv Ment Dis 178:392–395, 1990

Reboul J, Schuller E, Pialoux G, et al: Immunoglobulins and complement components in 37 patients infected by HIV-1 virus: comparison of general (systemic) and intrathecal immunity. J Neurol Sci 89:243–252, 1989

Wiley CA, Masliah E, Morey M, et al: Neocortical damage during HIV infection. Ann Neurol 29:651–657, 1991

CHAPTER 2 4

Neuropsychiatric Aspects of Rheumatic Disease

Select the single best response for each question.

24.1 Systemic lupus erythematosus (SLE) is considered the prototypical autoimmune disease. Which of the following is true regarding the neuropsychiatric symptoms in SLE?

A. The American College of Rheumatology criteria for neurological disorders include dementia, psychosis, and seizures.

B. Inflammatory cells in the cerebral vessel walls are seen in the majority of cases, implicating central nervous system (CNS) vasculitis as the mechanism for neuropsychiatric symptoms.

C. Lupus commonly presents with primarily neuropsychiatric symptoms.

D. Contemporary studies with systematized methodology have validated that psychosis is common in SLE.

E. Suicidal behavior in SLE has been correlated with active disease and abnormal electroencephalogram (EEG).

The correct response is option E.

The occurrence of suicide in lupus patients was found to be associated with active disease and a diffusely slow EEG.

The American College of Rheumatology criteria for neurological disorders is limited to psychosis and seizures. The major pathological finding in lupus is microinfarction associated with necrosis of small vessels, whereas inflammatory cells in the cerebral vessel walls are rarely seen. Lupus uncommonly presents with neuropsychiatric features, whereas CNS events often occur early in the course of the disease. Psychotic states in lupus have not been well characterized, and in recent studies using modern standardized assessments and diagnostic criteria, psychosis is unusual. **(pp. 814–818)**

24.2 Neuropsychiatric diagnosis in SLE may be challenging because of the multiplicity of symptoms and variably progressive nature of the illness. Which of the following is true?

A. Cognitive deficits (on neuropsychological examination) have been reported in one-half of SLE patients without previous CNS disease.

B. Cognitive impairment in SLE is closely correlated to white matter disease on magnetic resonance imaging (MRI).

C. Cognitive impairment in SLE has been correlated to the presence of antiphospholipid antibody.

D. MRI generally reveals periventricular, rather than subcortical white-matter lesions, which assists in differentiation from multiple sclerosis.

E. MRI findings are rare in SLE patients without CNS symptoms.

The correct response is option C.

Several studies demonstrated correlation between cognitive impairment and the presence of antiphospholipid antibody. Cognitive impairments have been reported in 35% of patients without previous CNS disease. MRI evidence of white-matter abnormalities has not been correlated to cognitive impairment in SLE. MRI generally reveals subcortical rather than preventricular lesions. MRI abnormalities are commonly seen in lupus patients with no history of cerebral involvement. **(pp. 818–819)**

24.3 Which of the following is true regarding Sjögren's syndrome?

A. Cortical dementia is a common neuropsychiatric finding.
B. The Minnesota Multiphasic Personality Inventory (MMPI) scales of hypochondriasis, depression, and hysteria have been found to be elevated in patients with Sjögren's syndrome.
C. Whereas parkinsonism is reported in patients with Sjögren's syndrome, it is no more common than in other rheumatic illnesses.
D. MRI reveals white- and gray-matter hyperintensities only in symptomatic patients.
E. Serum antineuronal antibodies may be found but do not correlate to presence or absence of neuropsychiatric symptoms.

The correct response is option B.

The MMPI scales of hypochondriasis, depression, and hysteria are elevated in patients with Sjögren's syndrome.

MRI reveals multiple small white- and gray-matter T2 hyperintensities in both symptomatic and asymptomatic patients. Subcortical dementia has been described in patients with Sjögren's syndrome, but cortical dementia has not been found. Parkinsonism stands out as distinctive for Sjögren's syndrome among the rheumatic disorders. Serum antineuronal antibodies are significantly more common in patients with Sjögren's syndrome with major neurological complications than in those without such findings. **(pp. 822–823)**

24.4 A middle-aged male presents with fever, weight loss, hypertension, fatigue, purpura, ulcers, headache, and livedo reticularis. On examination, psychosis, confusion, and cognitive impairment are noted. A likely diagnosis is

A. Polyarteritis nodosa.
B. Takayasu's arteritis.
C. Giant cell arteritis.
D. Wegener's granulomatosis.
E. Churg-Strauss syndrome.

The correct response is option A.

Polyarteritis nodosa is most common in middle-age men, Takayasu's arteritis mostly affects young women, and giant cell arteritis is a disease of late life, with a female predominance. Wegener's granulomatosis' peak incidence is in late midlife; Churg-Strauss syndrome is primarily a disease of early adult life, but it can occur at any age. **(pp. 823–824)**

24.5   Corticosteroids are a mainstay of treatment of autoimmune disease but may induce neuropsychiatric symptoms in their own right. Which of the following is true?

A. Neuropsychiatric syndromes are seen in more than 20% of patients following the use of corticosteroids as an idiosyncratic, rather than dose-dependent, phenomenon.
B. Neuropsychiatric symptoms occur early in the course of treatment and disappear when treatment is over, without a withdrawal syndrome.
C. Prior history of mood disorder profoundly increases the risk of corticosteroid-induced mood disorder.
D. Steroid dementia is a relatively common syndrome among corticosteroid-induced neuropsychiatric syndromes.
E. Antipsychotic medications should be used to counter corticosteroid-induced psychotic symptoms.

The correct response is option E.

Antipsychotic medications may be used to counter psychotic symptoms induced by corticosteroid treatment.

Psychiatric syndromes were seen in only 5.7% of patients treated with glucocorticoids (Lewis and Smith 1983). The psychiatric symptoms characteristically appear early in the course of treatment and disappear rapidly when treatment is discontinued, although symptoms may also occur as part of a glucocorticoid withdrawal syndrome (Wolkowitz et al. 1997). Prior history of mood disorder does not appear to increase the risk of corticosteroid-induced mood disorder (Wolkowitz et al. 1993). Steroid dementia is rarely seen. **(pp. 831–832)**

References

Lewis DA, Smith RE: Steroid-induced psychiatric syndromes: a report of 14 cases and a review of the literature. J Affect Disord 5:319–332, 1983
Wolkowitz OM, Coppola R, Breier A, et al: Quantitative electroencephalographic correlates of steroid administration in man. Neuropsychobiology 27:224–230, 1993
Wolkowitz O, Reus VI, Canick J, et al: Glucocorticoid medication, memory and steroid psychosis in medical illness. Ann N Y Acad Sci 823:81–96, 1997

C H A P T E R   2 5

Neuropsychiatric Aspects of Endocrine Disorders

Select the single best response for each question.

25.1   Insulin-dependent diabetes mellitus (IDDM) is in many ways the prototypical metabolic disorder with substantial neuropsychiatric comorbidity. Which of the following is true regarding the neuropsychiatric aspects of diabetes mellitus?

A.   Impaired performance on visuospatial tasks is associated with children who develop diabetes mellitus before the age of 5 years, compared with children with an older age at onset.

B.   Symptomatic hypoglycemia episodes are correlated with abnormal neuropsychological test performance, but asymptomatic hypoglycemia episodes are not.

C.   Degree of chronic metabolic control (based on measurements of glycosylated hemoglobin) has not been correlated to neuropsychological test performance.

D.   The prevalence of depression in diabetes is much higher than in other chronic diseases.

E.   When symptoms of depression that may be attributed to the diabetic condition are excluded from a diagnosis of a mood disorder, the prevalence of depression in diabetic patients is decreased by 50%.

The correct response is option A.

Children with early-onset IDDM score lower on visuospatial tasks than other diabetic patients and sibling control subjects (Rovet et al. 1987).

    Both asymptomatic and symptomatic hypoglycemia is associated with deficits in neuropsychological performance. Degree of chronic metabolic control has been correlated to neuropsychological impairment. Carney's (1998) review of studies of prevalence of depression in diabetes emphasized that depression in diabetes is no more prevalent than depression in other chronic diseases. When symptoms of depression that may be attributed to the diabetic condition are excluded from a diagnosis of mood disorder, the prevalence of depression in diabetic patients was decreased from 36% to 32.5%. **(pp. 852–853)**

25.2   Management of depression in diabetic patients may be of great importance in facilitating medical compliance and self-care. Which of the following is true regarding management of depression in diabetic patients?

A.   In both IDDM and non-insulin-dependent diabetes mellitus (NIDDM), the diabetic condition predates the onset of depressive symptoms.

B.   A depressed state correlates with increased insulin resistance in some patients.

C.   Depression has been associated with an increased risk of diabetic retinopathy in NIDDM (type II) diabetes but not in IDDM (type I) diabetes.

D.   Because of their risk of increased appetite and blood glucose, tricyclic antidepressants (TCAs) should be avoided in diabetic patients with neuropathic pain.

E. Despite their tendency to modestly increase serum glucose levels, selective serotonin reuptake inhibitors (SSRIs) are preferred for depressed diabetic patients because of their overall greater safety in these patients.

The correct response is option B.

Depression correlates with increased insulin resistance in some patients.

In patients with NIDDM, the depressive symptoms appear to precede the development of diabetes, whereas in patients with IDDM, the diabetic presentation precedes that of the depressive phenomenology (Lustman et al. 1988). In a 10-year prospective study, depression was found to be one of three factors independently associated with the onset of diabetic retinopathy in 24 children with IDDM (Kovacs et al. 1997). Monoamine oxidase inhibitors tend to exacerbate hypoglycemia and are associated with significant weight gain. TCAs are associated with marked increases in appetite, body weight, and blood glucose. SSRIs are associated with modest reductions in serum glucose and body weight, and as such they are the first-line antidepressants of choice in treating diabetic patients. **(pp. 853–855)**

25.3 Hypothyroidism serves as a model for neuropsychiatric symptoms directly attributable to a metabolic illness. Which of the following is true?

A. Because of the physical lethargy experienced by hypothyroid patients, anxiety symptoms are rare, in less than 5%.
B. The most severe cognitive manifestation in hypothyroidism is dementia.
C. Replacement of thyroid hormone in the form of T_3 (rather than T_4) has a specific effect on improving depressed mood but a negligible effect on cognitive performance.
D. Mood disorders, typically depression, have been found in 50% of patients with hypothyroidism.
E. Psychotic symptoms are the second most common group of neuropsychiatric illnesses in unselected hypothyroid populations.

The correct response is option D.

Depression is the second most frequent syndrome in hypothyroid patients, found in about 50% of patients.

Anxiety occurs in approximately 30% of patients. The most severe cognitive manifestation of hypothyroidism is delirium. Replacement of thyroid hormone in the form of T_3 has specific effects on both mood and cognition and is thus preferred to T_4. Although psychosis is the most common psychiatric symptom in hypothyroidism, it represents only 5% of the psychiatric morbidity in unselected samples. **(pp. 855–857)**

25.4 Because of advances in analysis of thyroid function and greater appreciation of the neuropsychiatric correlates of various thyroid disturbances, a system of grading has been developed. A patient who exhibits elevated thyroid-stimulating hormone (TSH), normal thyroid hormone levels, exaggerated TSH response to thyrotropin-releasing hormone (TRH), and increased risk of major depression that responds poorly to antidepressants would be said to have which grade of hypothyroidism?

A. Grade I.
B. Grade II.
C. Grade III.
D. Grade IV.
E. Grade V.

The correct response is option B.

Grade II. Grade I is defined by low levels of thyroid hormones and an elevated TSH concentration. Grade III is characterized by an exaggerated TSH response to TRH in the setting of normal basal TSH, T_3, and T_4 levels. Grade IV is characterized by antithyroid antibodies in the serum but with normal circulating basal TSH and T_4 levels and a normal TRH stimulation test. **(pp. 857–858)**

25.5   Hyperthyroidism has also been associated with a specific range of neuropsychiatric symptoms and syndromes. Which of the following is true?
   A. Because of the degree of systemic metabolic disturbances in hyperthyroidism, the majority of patients exhibit psychopathology as a result of hyperthyroidism.
   B. In studies of both selected and unselected hyperthyroidism patients, anxiety disorders are the most common neuropsychiatric illnesses.
   C. Cognitive disturbance in hyperthyroidism is as common as it is in hypothyroidism.
   D. In hyperthyroid patients with depressive symptoms, the physical symptoms of hyperthyroidism precede mood symptoms in the vast majority of cases.
   E. In hyperthyroidism, both mania and psychosis are rare.

The correct response is option E.

Mania or hypomania and psychosis are uncommon in hyperthyroid patients, occurring in only about 2.1% of unselected cases.

Serious psychopathology only occurs in a minority of patients. Major depression is the most common psychiatric manifestation; however, the mood symptoms may precede the development of physical signs and symptoms of hyperthyroidism in some patients. The prevalence of cognitive disturbance in hyperthyroidism is considerably less than that in hypothyroidism. **(pp. 858–860)**

25.6   In Cushing's syndrome, which of the following is true regarding neuropsychiatric comorbidity?
   A. Mania, simulating bipolar disorder, is seen as commonly as is depression.
   B. The most common neuropsychiatric presentation in Cushing's syndrome is a mixed profile of anxiety and depression.
   C. Treatment of the hormonal disturbance in Cushing's syndrome rarely reverses mood symptoms without concurrent antidepressants.
   D. Delirium is common in Cushing's syndrome and is the most likely cause of psychotic symptoms.
   E. Cognitive impairment, usually of a moderate degree, is common in Cushing's syndrome.

The correct response is option B.

Mixed anxiety and depressive symptoms are the most common psychiatric manifestation of Cushing's syndrome (Loosen et al. 1992; Mazet et al. 1981).

Mania is rarely reported. Treating Cushing's syndrome has been shown to improve the mood disorder in most patients. Psychosis and delirium are rarely reported in the Cushing's disease literature. Cognitive impairment has been relatively infrequently reported, and, when documented, it has been mild. **(pp. 861–864)**

25.7   Parathyroid disease, although relatively uncommon, has been associated with neuropsychiatric illnesses. Which of the following is true?

   A. Neuropsychiatric symptoms tend to be stereotypical irrespective of the serum calcium level.
   B. Psychiatric symptoms tend to remain persistent despite parathyroidectomy.
   C. Mood disorders are the most common neuropsychiatric disturbance in hypoparathyroidism.
   D. The risk and types of neuropsychiatric symptoms in hypoparathyroidism are the same for idiopathic and surgical types.
   E. Correction of serum calcium levels in hypoparathyroidism has been found to improve neuropsychiatric symptoms.

The correct response is option E.

Correction of serum calcium levels in hypoparathyroidism has been found to improve neuropsychiatric symptoms. Preoperative symptoms of psychological distress improved within 1 month after removal of the parathyroid adenoma. Cognitive disorders are the most frequently encountered syndromes in hypoparathyroidism. The risks and types of neuropsychiatric symptoms vary between patients with surgical hypoparathyroidism and those with the idiopathic form. Intellectual dysfunction and delirium are more common in patients with surgical hypoparathyroidism. Depressive, psychotic, and anxiety symptoms are more common in the surgical group than in the idiopathic group. **(pp. 866–868)**

References

Carney C: Diabetes mellitus and major depressive disorder: an overview of prevalence, complications, and treatment. Depression and Anxiety 7:149–157, 1998

Kovacs M, Obrosky DS, Goldstone D, et al: Major depressive disorder in youth with IDDM: a controlled prospective study of course and outcome. Diabetes Care 20:45–51, 1997

Loosen PT, Chambliss R, DeBold CR, et al: Psychiatric phenomenology in Cushing's disease. Pharmacopsychiatry 25:192–198, 1992

Lustman PJ, Griffith LS, Clouse RE: Depression in adults with diabetes: results of a 5-year follow-up study. Diabetes Care 11:605–612, 1988

Mazet P, Simon D, Luton J-P, et al: Syndrome de Cushing: symptomatologie psychique et personnalite de 50 malades. Nouvelle Presse Medicale 10:2565–2570, 1981

Rovet JF, Ehrlich RM, Hoppe M: Intellectual deficits associated with early onset of insulin-dependent diabetes mellitus in children. Diabetes Care 10:510–515, 1987

C H A P T E R   2 6

Neuropsychiatric Aspects of Poisons and Toxins

Select the single best response for each question.

26.1 Aluminum is a ubiquitous metal with numerous industrial and medical applications. Unfortunately, aluminum poisoning may result in substantial neuropsychiatric pathology. Which of the following is true regarding aluminum poisoning?

    A. Aluminum is readily absorbed via the gastrointestinal tract, with intraluminal pH having a negligible role in degree of absorption.

    B. Patients with acute renal failure often have a precipitous onset of dialysis encephalopathy, featuring personality changes and psychotic symptoms.

    C. Dementia due to aluminum toxicity in dialysis patients characteristically features disturbed concentration, attention, orientation, and memory.

    D. Electroencephalographic changes in aluminum-toxicity dementia are only seen after the onset of cognitive symptoms.

    E. Despite characteristic electroencephalographic abnormalities, seizures and myoclonic jerks are not typical clinical findings.

The correct response is option C.

Dementia due to aluminum toxicity in dialysis patients manifests gradually as disturbances of concentration, attention, orientation, and memory.

    Aluminum is poorly absorbed through the gastrointestinal tract, although, depending on intraluminal pH, absorption can range from 0.0005% to 24%. Patients with chronic renal failure on long-term dialysis can develop dialysis encephalopathy, characterized by gradual development of personality changes and visual and auditory hallucinations. Electroencephalographic abnormalities may precede the onset of cognitive symptoms. Myoclonic jerks and tonic-clonic seizures can also occur with a high incidence. **(pp. 878–881)**

26.2 Arsenic is an element associated with many industrial processes. Which of the following is true regarding arsenic poisoning and its neuropsychiatric manifestations?

    A. Arsenic localizes in the erythrocytes and platelets but not in leukocytes.

    B. Neuropsychiatric manifestations of arsenic poisoning are a direct result of its ability to readily penetrate the blood-brain barrier.

    C. Acute exposure to arsenic typically produces visual disturbances.

    D. Laboratory methods for arsenic analysis include hair analysis to assess both acute and long-term exposure.

    E. Seizures, muscle spasms, and muscular twitching may follow acute exposure.

The correct response is option E.

Neuropsychiatric symptoms of acute arsenic poisoning include spasms, muscular twitching, and seizures.

Arsenic localizes in the erythrocytes and leukocytes. Long-term exposure to arsenic may result in visual disturbances. Although there is minimal penetration of the blood-brain barrier, arsenic readily crosses the placenta and may produce fetal damage (Klaassen 1990). The human sample of choice for arsenic analysis is urine for recent exposure and hair for long-term exposure. **(p. 881)**

26.3   Lead and manganese poisoning are associated with characteristic neuropsychiatric symptoms. Which of the following is true?

A.   Clinical symptoms of lead poisoning emerge at blood levels of 400 mg/L in both children and adults.
B.   The first recognizable symptoms of lead poisoning are headaches, tremor, and seizures.
C.   Seizures caused by lead toxicity are generalized, not focal, and respond to antiepileptic medications.
D.   Manganese toxicity features a sequence of neuropsychiatric disturbances, progressing from mood and psychotic symptoms, to parkinsonian motor symptoms, and finally to frank dystonias and chorea.
E.   Blood and urinary manganese levels correlate well with degree of clinical symptoms.

The correct response is option D.

Manganese intoxication is characterized by mood changes, emotional lability, auditory and visual hallucinations, and neuropsychological impairment. It may progress to a parkinsonian disorder and to dystonia and chorea.

Clinical symptoms of lead poisoning in adults appear when blood levels reach approximately 400 mg/L but do so at much lower levels in children. The first recognizable symptoms of lead poisoning are fatigue, bradyphrenia, memory impairment, dyssomnia, and anxiety. Seizures caused by lead toxicity are generalized or focal and are refractory to medication. Urinary manganese concentration does not correlate with changes in clinical neurologic status; however, urinary manganese does indicate recent exposure (Cook et al. 1974; Roels et al. 1987). **(pp. 882–883)**

26.4   Mercury poisoning may be a particularly serious problem in certain high-risk occupations. Which of the following is true regarding mercury poisoning?

A.   Elemental mercury is particularly dangerous because it is readily absorbed both by inhalation and ingestion.
B.   Organic mercury, such as alkyl mercury, is lipid soluble and profoundly neurotoxic.
C.   Exposure to inhaled elemental mercury leads to characteristic neuropsychiatric symptoms such as coarse tremor, increased energy, hypersexuality, and mania.
D.   Dentists exposed to organic mercury have been found to have decreased motor speed and visual scanning with preserved concentration, memory, and coordination.
E.   Methylmercury poisoning is associated with headache, irritability, and depression, and is treated with British anti-Lewisite (BAL).

The correct response is option B.

Organic mercury, particularly alkyl mercury, is lipid soluble, well absorbed through the gastrointestinal tract, and has substantial neurotoxicity.

Mercury in elemental form is a liquid that vaporizes easily and is well absorbed by inhalation but poorly absorbed through the gastrointestinal tract. Exposure to inhaled elemental mercury leads to insomnia, nervousness, mild tremor, headache, emotional lability, fatigue, decreased sexual drive, depression, and impaired cognition, judgment, and coordination (Louria 1988). Dentists exposed to organic mercury have significant deficits in motor speed, visual scanning, concentration, memory, and coordination. Methylmercury poisoning is associated with headache, sleep disturbances, dizziness, irritability, emotional instability, mania, and depression (Elhassani 1983); treatment with BAL is contraindicated because it has been shown to increase methylmercury levels in laboratory animals (Klaassen 1990). **(p. 883)**

26.5 Carbon monoxide poisoning is often encountered in suicide attempts. Which of the following is true regarding the neuropsychiatric implications of carbon monoxide poisoning?

A. Acute exposure to carbon monoxide results in disorientation to time and place but not to person.
B. A brief recovery period following exposure may be followed by cognitive, psychotic, and mood symptoms 2–4 weeks later.
C. The greater affinity of hemoglobin for carbon monoxide than for oxygen (approximately 20 times greater) accounts for the potency of carbon monoxide as a poison.
D. The most common symptoms in the delayed neuropsychiatric syndrome of carbon monoxide poisoning include apathy, disorientation, amnesia, and delusions.
E. The electroencephalogram (EEG) is a valuable predictive test because patients with markedly abnormal EEGs do not recover substantially.

The correct response is option B.

After 2–4 weeks, a sudden deterioration may develop, consisting of amnestic disturbances, disorientation, signs of dementia, hypokinesia, bizarre and occasionally psychotic behavior, urinary incontinence, personality changes, apathy, emotional instability, anxiety, and autonomic dysregulation (Min 1986).

Acute exposure to carbon monoxide results in disorientation to time, place, and person. The affinity of hemoglobin for carbon monoxide is 200 times greater than that for oxygen, thus accounting for the potency and lethality of carbon monoxide. The most common neuropsychiatric symptoms in delayed syndrome associated with carbon monoxide poisoning include apathy, disorientation, amnesia, hypokinesia, and mutism. EEGs are not thought to have much predictive value because patients with markedly abnormal EEGs may show complete recovery (Ellenhorn 1997). **(pp. 885–886)**

26.6 Which of the following is true regarding neuropsychiatric manifestations of organophosphate intoxication?

A. Organophosphates are environmentally problematic because of their propensity to resist rapid degradation.
B. Mild exposure to organophosphates produces anxiety, restlessness, dry mouth, dryness of the conjunctivae, and pupillary mydriasis.
C. Moderate exposure to organophosphates leads to tremors, depression, tachycardia, hypotonia, and seizures.
D. The onset of symptoms from organophosphate toxicity is rapid (within several minutes), irrespective of route of exposure.
E. Neuropsychiatric symptoms such as depression, fatigue, anxiety, and irritability may persist for 1 year following exposure to organophosphates.

The correct response is option E.

Neuropsychiatric symptoms of depression, fatigue, anxiety, and irritability may be long lasting and persist for as long as 1 year. Organophosphates are degraded fairly rapidly. Mild exposure to organophosphates produces weakness, headache, dizziness, nausea, salivation, lacrimation, miosis, and moderate bronchial spasm. Moderate exposure leads to abrupt weakness, visual disturbances, excessive salivation, sweating, vomiting, diarrhea, bradycardia, hypertonia, tremors, impaired gait, miosis, chest pain, and cyanosis of mucous membranes. The onset of action of organophosphates is dependent on the type and the route of exposure. **(pp. 880, Table 26–5, and 889)**

References

Cook DG, Fahn S, Brait KA: Chronic manganese intoxication. Arch Neurol 30:59–64, 1974

Elhassani SB: The many faces of methylmercury poisoning. J Toxicol Clin Toxicol 19:875–906, 1983

Ellenhorn MJ: Ellenhorn's Medical Toxicology: Diagnosis and Treatment of Human Poisoning. Baltimore, MD, Williams & Wilkins, 1997

Klaassen CD: Heavy metals and heavy-metal antagonists, in Goodman and Gilman's The Pharmacological Basis of Therapeutics, 8th Edition. Edited by Goodman-Gilman A, Rall TA, Nies AS, et al. New York, Pergamon, 1990, pp 1592–1614

Louria DB: Trace metal poisoning, in Cecil Textbook of Medicine. Edited by Wyngaarden JB, Smith LHJ. Philadelphia, PA, WB Saunders, 1988, pp 2385–2393

Min SK: A brain syndrome associated with delayed neuropsychiatric sequelae following acute carbon monoxide intoxication. Acta Psychiatr Scand 73:80–86, 1986

Roels H, Lauwerys R, Genet P, et al: Relationship between external and internal parameters of exposure to manganese in workers from a manganese oxide and salt producing plant. Am J Ind Med 11:297–305, 1987

C H A P T E R 2 7

Neuropsychiatric Aspects of Ethanol and Other Chemical Dependencies

Select the single best response for each question.

27.1 The substance-related phenomenon of specific physical and/or behavioral/motivational disturbances that present when a drug is discontinued or reduced in dose is referred to as

A. Tolerance.
B. Sensitization.
C. Reverse tolerance.
D. Dependence.
E. Withdrawal.

The correct response is option E.

Withdrawal. *Tolerance* is the weakening of a drug effect after repeated use. *Sensitization* or *reverse tolerance* is the stronger effect produced by a drug after repeated use. *Dependence* is the need for continued drug exposure to avoid a withdrawal syndrome. **(pp. 899–900)**

27.2 Which of the following drugs acts by the stimulation of monoamine release?

A. Opiates.
B. Cocaine.
C. Amphetamine.
D. Hallucinogens.
E. Phencyclidine (PCP).

The correct response is option C.

Amphetamine stimulates monoamine release. **(p. 901, Table 27–1)**

27.3 The locus coeruleus has been implicated in mechanisms of substance dependence. Which of the following is true?

A. Inhibition of the locus coeruleus is the cause of the physical symptoms of opiate withdrawal.
B. The acute effects of opiates on locus coeruleus neurons occur via direct effects on the K^+ channel and Na^+ current.
C. Tolerance, withdrawal, and dependence are in part mediated by upregulation of the cyclic adenosine monophosphate (cAMP) pathway in locus coeruleus neurons.

D. Long-term opiate administration is associated with inhibition of norepinephrine synthesis.

E. Administration of glutamate receptor antagonists into the locus coeruleus stimulates its activity in opiate withdrawal.

The correct response is option C.

Tolerance, dependence, and withdrawal are mediated in part via upregulation of the cAMP pathway as a compensatory adaptation to long-term exposure to opiate.

Overactivation of locus coeruleus neurons is both necessary and sufficient for producing many behavioral signs of opiate withdrawal. Opiates activate the K^+ channel and inhibit the Na^+ current. Norepinephrine synthesis is increased after long-term opiate administration. Administration of glutamate receptor antagonists into the cerebral ventricles or the locus coeruleus attenuates activation of locus coeruleus neurons during opiate withdrawal. **(pp. 903–905)**

27.4 Regarding the phenomenon of "priming" in drug abuse (wherein a small reexposure to an abused drug leads to relapse), which of the following is *not* true?

A. Priming has been demonstrated for both opiates and psychostimulants.

B. Cross-priming refers to opiates being used to prime relapse into abuse of psychostimulants.

C. Priming injections of opiates and psychostimulants into the nucleus accumbens (NA) induce relapse into opioid-seeking behavior in animals.

D. Infusions of opioids into brain regions rich in opioid receptors produce a vigorous increase in drug-seeking behavior.

E. Dopamine antagonists block the priming effects of opioids and psychostimulants.

The correct response is option D.

Infusions of opioids into brain regions rich in opioid receptors are ineffective at inducing relapse to drug-seeking behavior.

The priming effect has been demonstrated for both opiates and psychostimulants. Opiates such as morphine can trigger relapse to cocaine-seeking behavior, known as "cross-priming." Priming injections of opiates and psychostimulants into the nucleus accumbens induce relapse to heroin-seeking behavior. Dopamine antagonists can block the priming effects of heroin, amphetamine, and cocaine. **(pp. 907–908)**

27.5 Psychosocial stress is commonly associated with relapse into drug abuse. Which of the following is true?

A. In animals, stress-induced relapse into heroin-seeking behavior requires physical dependence.

B. Stress-induced heroin-seeking behavior in animals is fully attenuated by pretreatment with dopamine antagonists.

C. Stress activates the prefrontal cortex and inhibits the pathway from the frontal cortex to dopamine neurons in the ventral tegmental area (VTA).

D. Drug-withdrawal states readily induce drug-seeking behavior in animals.

E. Activation of D_2, D_3, and D_4 receptors in rats induces relapse in cocaine-seeking behavior.

The correct response is option E.

Activation of D_2, D_3, and D_4 receptors induces a profound and prolonged relapse to cocaine-seeking behavior in rats (De Vries et al. 1999; Self et al. 1996).

Stress-induced relapse to heroin-seeking behavior is not tied to physical dependence on heroin. Stress-induced relapse in animals is partially attenuated by pretreatment with dopamine antagonists (Shaham and Stewart 1996). Stress activates the prefrontal cortex and activates the pathway from the prefrontal cortex to dopamine neurons in the VTA. In animal models, drug withdrawal–like processes fail to induce relapse to drug-seeking behavior. **(pp. 909–910)**

27.6   Various structural changes have been described in the VTA and the NA in response to long-term treatment with morphine, cocaine, or alcohol. Which of the following is *not* true after long-term substance exposure?

   A. Tyrosine hydroxylase levels are increased in the VTA.
   B. Tyrosine hydroxylase levels are decreased in the NA.
   C. Neurofilament levels are decreased in the VTA.
   D. The size of VTA dopamine neurons is decreased.
   E. There is an increase in axoplasmic transport from the VTA to the NA.

The correct response is option E.

Morphine causes a reduction in axoplasmic transport from the VTA to the NA. **(pp. 912–914)**

References

De Vries TJ, Schoffelmeer ANM, Binnekade R, et al: Dopaminergic mechanisms mediating the incentive to seek cocaine and heroin following long-term withdrawal of IV drug self-administration. Psychopharmacology (Berl) 143:254–260, 1999

Self DW, Barnhart WJ, Lehman DA, et al: Opposite modulation of cocaine-seeking behavior by D1-like and D2-like dopamine receptor agonists. Science 271:1586–1589, 1996

Shaham Y, Stewart J: Effects of opioid and dopamine receptor antagonists on relapse induced by stress and re-exposure to heroin in rats. Psychopharmacology (Berl) 125:385–391, 1996

C H A P T E R 2 8

Neuropsychiatric Aspects of Dementias Associated With Motor Dysfunction

Select the single best response for each question.

28.1 Which of the following is true regarding dementia due to Huntington's disease?

A. Aphasia is prominent.
B. Positron emission tomography (PET) studies demonstrate hypometabolism in the caudate nucleus.
C. Degeneration begins in the anterior caudate nucleus and proceeds posteriorly.
D. Severity of motor symptoms is independent of the emotional state.
E. Degeneration of the frontal lobes correlates more closely with deficits in executive functions than does degeneration of the caudate nucleus.

The correct response is option B.

PET studies demonstrate glucose hypometabolism in the caudate nucleus.

Most patients with dementia due to Huntington's disease have nonaphasic dementia. Degeneration begins in the medial caudate nucleus and proceeds laterally to the putamen and occasionally to the globus pallidus. Severity of motor symptoms is often influenced by emotional states. Atrophy of the caudate nucleus is generally more strongly correlated than measures of frontal atrophy. **(pp. 925–927)**

28.2 Specific neuropsychiatric findings (some of which require elucidation by formal neuropsychological examination) of dementia due to Huntington's disease typically include which one of the following?

A. Early loss of language functions.
B. Greater impairment in recognition than retrieval memory.
C. Anomia.
D. Defects in planning, organizing, and mental flexibility.
E. Lack of awareness of cognitive deficits.

The correct response is option D.

Planning, organizing, and mental flexibility are affected early in Huntington's disease. In patients with Huntington's disease, language functions are relatively preserved and object naming is relatively preserved even in advanced cases. There is greater impairment in information retrieval than in recognition memory. Awareness of deficits is present, but judgment is poor. **(pp. 928–929)**

28.3   Which of the following is true regarding dementia due to Parkinson's disease?

    A. There is a high concordance rate for identical twins, suggesting strong genetic factors.

    B. Neuronal loss in the nucleus basalis of Meynert is a typical finding in both idiopathic and postencephalitic Parkinson's disease with dementia.

    C. Because dementia due to Parkinson's disease is a subcortical dementia, visuospatial impairment is rare.

    D. Executive function deficits are common.

    E. Communication difficulties in dementia due to Parkinson's disease are caused solely by dysarthria, not language difficulties.

The correct response is option D.

Executive function deficits are quite common and include verbal and visual deficits, visuospatial impairments, executive dysfunctions, and language difficulties.

    A low concordance rate has been reported in identical twins, thus disproving a strong genetic factor. Neuronal loss in the nucleus basalis of Meynert is common with idiopathic Parkinson's disease but not with postencephalitic Parkinson's disease. A large body of literature exists describing problems in visuospatial impairment, including spatial capacities, facial recognition, body schema, pursuit tracking, spatial attention, visual analysis, and judgments concerning position in space. Communication difficulties in Parkinson's disease are mostly caused by speech abnormalities such as hypophonia and dysarthria. However, language impairments also occur. **(pp. 931–933)**

28.4   Which of the following is true regarding the diagnosis and management of noncognitive neuropsychiatric symptoms in dementia due to Parkinson's disease?

    A. Mood disorders are more common in late-onset cases.

    B. Atypical depression in Parkinson's disease features reversed neurovegetative signs rather than anxiety.

    C. Medications are the most common cause of psychotic symptoms in Parkinson's disease.

    D. Dopamine agonists and anticholinergics effectively treat postural instability.

    E. Selegiline may be safely combined with low-dose selective serotonin reuptake inhibitors (SSRIs) in Parkinson's disease.

The correct response is option C.

Most authors believe that medications are the most common cause of psychosis in Parkinson's disease.

    Mood disorders are more common in early onset cases. Atypical depression with predominant anxiety also occurs. Dopamine agonists and anticholinergic agents can effectively treat rigidity, bradykinesia, and tremor, but postural instability is resistant to the effects of drugs. Selegiline combined with an SSRI may produce hypertensive crises. **(pp. 933–935)**

28.5   Dementia with Lewy bodies (DLB) is an increasingly appreciated form of dementia, with a characteristic pattern of neuropsychiatric symptoms. Which of the following is true regarding DLB?

    A. Visual hallucinations, usually unformed and fleeting, are common early in the course of DLB.

    B. Fluctuations in cognitive performance, but not level of consciousness, are characteristic.

    C. Depression is less common in DLB than in other types of dementia.

    D. Greater frontal lobe atrophy in DLB reliably differentiates DLB from Alzheimer's disease.

    E. DLB patients tend to respond as well as or better than Alzheimer's disease patients to cholinesterase inhibitors.

The correct response is option E.

DLB patients may respond as well or better to cholinesterase inhibitors than patients with Alzheimer's disease (Fergusson and Howard 2000).

Visual hallucinations are persistent and well formed. Fluctuating consciousness is one of the interesting clinical features of DLB. Depression is more common in DLB than in other types of dementia. Whereas more frontal lobe atrophy has been found in DLB, there is an insufficient difference to make a clinical differentiation in diagnosis. **(p. 936)**

28.6   Which of the following is true regarding progressive supranuclear palsy (PSP)?

A. Smooth pursuit eye movements are affected before saccadic eye movements.
B. Severe dementia early in the illness is typical.
C. Aphasia, apraxia, and agnosia are prominent symptoms.
D. Forced, inappropriate expressions of crying, laughter, or rage are typical.
E. Because of the presence of parkinsonian symptoms in PSP, levodopa treatment is generally successful for motor symptoms.

The correct response is option D.

Forced inappropriate crying or laughing with outbursts of rage is common in progressive supranuclear palsy, or Steele-Richardson-Olszewski syndrome.

The earliest eye movement abnormalities include loss of vertical saccade velocity. Not all patients with PSP have noticeable dementia, and dementia is often not severe early in the course of PSP. Aphasia, apraxia, and agnosia are absent. Levodopa treatment is generally not successful. **(pp. 937–938)**

28.7   Which of the following is true of Fahr's disease?

A. Fahr's disease is a rare, inherited, autosomal recessive disorder.
B. Calcification (evident on neuroimaging) is restricted to the basal ganglia.
C. Patients typically present in early adulthood with dementia in the absence of mood or psychotic symptoms.
D. Apathy and memory impairments are prominent, with spared language functions.
E. Fahr's disease has been associated with hyperparathyroidism.

The correct response is option D.

Apathy, poor judgment, and memory impairment are prominent, and language function is often spared.

Fahr's disease is a rare inherited autosomal dominant disorder. Extensive calcification of the basal ganglia and periventricular white matter are evident on neuroimaging. Patients may present in early adulthood with a schizophrenia-like psychosis or mood disorder. Fahr's disease has been associated with hypoparathyroidism. **(p. 942)**

Reference

Fergusson E, Howard R: Donepezil for the treatment of psychosis in dementia with Lewy bodies. Int J Geriatr Psychiatry 15:280–281, 2000

C H A P T E R 2 9

Neuropsychiatric Aspects of Alzheimer's Disease and Other Dementing Illnesses

Select the single best response for each question.

29.1 Alzheimer's disease (AD) is the most common dementing illness in the United States and is associated with specific neuropathological findings and clinical neuropsychiatric symptoms. Which of the following is true?

A. The cortical degeneration in AD typically affects the primary motor and sensory cortex, whereas subcortical structures are spared.

B. Genes for amyloid precursor protein, presenilin 1 (PS1), and presenilin 2 (PS2) are all coded on chromosome 21, correlating with the much higher risk of AD in Down syndrome.

C. Because the apolipoprotein-E (APOE) ε4 allele is strongly correlated with early onset and more severe AD, it is presently recommended that asymptomatic individuals be screened for this gene.

D. The combination of APOE ε4 allele and head injury further increases the risk of subsequent AD.

E. Seizures early in the illness strongly suggest a diagnosis of AD.

The correct response is option D.

The presence of the ε4 variant of APOE combined with head trauma increases risk for AD eightfold (Nemetz et al. 1999).

Limbic, paralimbic, and cortical areas are maximally affected, whereas primary sensory and motor areas, thalamus, basal ganglia, and cerebellum are comparatively spared (Cummings and Benson 1992). Mutations in three genes produce the autosomal dominant form of AD: the amyloid precursor protein (APP) gene on chromosome 21, PS1 gene on chromosome 4, and PS2 gene on chromosome 1. The presence of APOE ε4 is neither necessary nor sufficient for the development of AD, thus routine testing for this gene in asymptomatic patients is not of value. Seizures early in the course of the illness usually suggest that a diagnosis of AD is unlikely. **(pp. 954–955)**

29.2   Which of the following is true regarding the neuropsychiatric symptoms in AD?

A. AD primarily is a diagnosis of exclusion and should be diagnosed presumptively after "reversible" dementias have been ruled out.

B. The cortical symptoms of apraxia and agnosia are commonly seen together in the early stages of the disease.

C. Verbal fluency and reading aloud by rote are lost early, whereas simple verbal repetition is preserved until late in the clinical course.

D. Personality changes are extremely common, and the usual personality manifestation is increased aggressiveness and disinhibition.

E. Delusions, including delusions of theft, infidelity, or abandonment, are present in up to 50% of AD patients.

The correct response is option E.

Delusions of theft, infidelity, abandonment, persecution, or a phantom boarder are present in up to 50% of patients with AD. Accurate diagnosis depends on a combination of inclusionary and exclusionary clinical features. Apraxia may be an early feature, whereas agnosia is associated with the later stages of the disease. Fluency of verbal output, repetition skills, and the ability to read aloud are retained until late in the disease. The most common personality change in AD is passivity or disengagement. **(pp. 955–956)**

29.3   Which of the following is true regarding the clinical and neuroimaging manifestations of AD?

A. Hallucinations, particularly auditory hallucinations, are seen in 50% of patients.

B. Mood symptoms are common in AD, and 40% of patients meet criteria for a major depressive episode.

C. Because of the risk of comorbid psychotic and depressive disorders, the risk of suicide in AD is high.

D. Studies with positron emission tomography with fluorodeoxyglucose (FDG-PET) reveal early loss of frontal lobe glucose utilization, followed by a later loss in the temporal lobes.

E. Magnetic resonance imaging (MRI) findings of hippocampal atrophy can be a sensitive early marker for AD.

The correct response is option E.

MRI findings reveal atrophy of the hippocampus and related structures early in the disease.

Hallucinations are not a common manifestation of AD. Few patients meet the criteria for major depressive disorder, but some elements of a depressive syndrome can occur in 20%–40% of patients with AD. Suicide is rare. FDG-PET studies early in the disease reveal diminished glucose utilization in the parietal lobes, followed by a later loss in the frontal lobes. **(pp. 956–957)**

29.4   Frontotemporal dementia (FTD) may come to the psychiatrist's attention because of the propensity for disorganized and/or disruptive behavior. Which of the following is true regarding FTD?

A. Age at onset for FTD is typically greater than 65 years.

B. Memory and visuospatial skills are degraded early, with relative preservation of language skills.

C. Approximately 15% of patients with amyotrophic lateral sclerosis develop FTD.

D. Because of the locus of neuropathology, naming deficits are rare.

E. As with AD, cholinergic neurons are preferentially affected in FTD.

The correct response is option C.

As many as 15% of patients with amyotrophic lateral sclerosis develop clinical symptoms consistent with FTD (Miller et al. 1994). Age at onset for FTD is typically between ages 40 and 65 years. Memory and visuospatial skills are relatively preserved, whereas naming deficits are prominent. Unlike with AD, in which cholinergic neurons are preferentially involved, no selective transmitter has been found for FTD. **(pp. 959–962)**

29.5 Vascular dementia is a common dementia syndrome that must often be differentiated from AD. Which of the following is true regarding vascular dementia?

   A. Motor symptoms of vascular dementia may include hyperreflexia, extensor plantar responses, and pseudobulbar palsy, whereas gait abnormalities are rare.
   B. Speech difficulties in vascular dementia are equally likely to result from aphasia and dysarthria.
   C. Because the neuropathology in vascular dementia is primarily subcortical, personality changes are rare.
   D. Severity of comorbid depression correlates strongly with degree of cognitive impairment in vascular dementia.
   E. MRI is preferable to computed tomography (CT) because of its superiority in imaging subcortical structures.

The correct response is option E.

MRI is more revealing than CT and demonstrates small subcortical infarctions and ischemic white-matter changes that are invisible on CT (Brown et al. 1988; Hershey et al. 1987).
   Motor findings of vascular dementia include weakness, spasticity, hyperreflexia, extensor plantar responses, bradykinesia, parkinsonism, and pseudobulbar palsy (Ishii et al. 1986). Gait abnormalities are also common. Speech and language assessments reveal dysarthria with relative preservation of language functions (Hier et al. 1985; Powell et al. 1988). Personality changes, depression, lability of mood, and delusions occur regularly. However, there is little relationship between the severity of depression and the degree of dementia (Cummings et al. 1987). **(pp. 973–976)**

29.6 Workup for reversible causes of dementia may reveal a correctable cause in up to 15% of patients. All of the following studies are included in a routine dementia assessment *except*

   A. Syphilis serology.
   B. Complete blood count (CBC).
   C. Vitamin B_{12}.
   D. Thyroid-stimulating hormone (TSH).
   E. Serum glucose.

The correct response is option A.

Routine tests include CBC, electrolytes, serum glucose, blood urea nitrogen, vitamin B_{12}, and TSH. Syphilis serology and tests for human immunodeficiency virus, Lyme disease, urinary tract infection (UTI), and heavy metal intoxication are optional (Knopman et al. 2001). **(p. 979)**

29.7   Dementia due to normal-pressure hydrocephalus (NPH) is potentially reversible. Numerous neuropsychiatric symptoms have been described in association with NPH. Which of the following is *not* typical of NPH?

   A. Aphasia, agnosia, and apraxia.
   B. Gait disturbance.
   C. Visuospatial disturbances.
   D. Impaired abstraction.
   E. Apathy.

The correct response is option A.

Aphasia, agnosia, and apraxia are absent or mild. Classic symptoms of NPH include dementia, gait disturbance, incontinence, visuospatial disturbances, and impaired abstraction and judgment. **(p. 976)**

References

Brown JJ, Hesselink JR, Rothrock JF: MR and CT of lacunar infarcts. American Journal of Radiology 151:367–372, 1988

Cummings JL, Benson DF: Dementia: A Clinical Approach. Boston, MA, Butterworth, 1992

Cummings JL, Miller B, Hill MA, et al: Neuropsychiatric aspects of multi-infarct dementia and dementia of the Alzheimer type. Arch Neurol 44(4):389–393, 1987

Hershey LA, Modic MT, Greenough G, et al: Magnetic resonance imaging in vascular dementia. Neurology 37:29–36, 1987

Hier DB, Hagenlocker K, Shindler AD: Language disintegration in dementia: effects of etiology and severity. Brain Lang 25:117–133, 1985

Ishii N, Nishihara Y, Imamura T: Why do frontal lobe symptoms predominate in vascular dementia with lacunes? Neurology 36:340–345, 1986

Knopman DS, DeKosky ST, Cummings JL, et al: Practice parameter: diagnosis of dementia (an evidence-based review). Report of the Quality Standards Subcommittee of the American Academy of Neurology. Neurology 56:1143–1153, 2001

Miller BL, Chang L, Oropilla G, et al: AD and frontal lobe dementias, in Textbook of Geriatric Neuropsychiatry. Edited by Coffey CE, Cummings JL. Washington, DC, American Psychiatric Press, 1994, pp 390–404

Nemetz PN, Leibson C, Naessens JM, et al: Traumatic brain injury and time to onset of AD: a population-based study. Am J Epidemiol 149(1):32–40, 1999

Powell AL, Cummings JL, Hill MA, et al: Speech and language alterations in multi-infarct dementia. Neurology 38:717–719, 1988

C H A P T E R   3 0

Neuropsychiatric Aspects of Schizophrenia

Select the single best response for each question.

30.1   The symptoms of schizophrenia have been classified as belonging to three major domains: 1) "positive" symptoms such as hallucinations and delusions, 2) thought disorder and bizarre behavior, and 3) "negative" symptoms such as anhedonia and poverty of thought. Which symptom was the most frequently reported psychotic symptom in the 1974 World Health Organization International Pilot Study of Schizophrenia?

    A. Lack of insight.
    B. Auditory hallucinations.
    C. Ideas of reference.
    D. Suspiciousness.
    E. Flatness of affect.

The correct response is option A.

The most frequent psychotic symptom in schizophrenia was lack of insight, in 97% of cases. Auditory hallucinations were the next most frequent symptom, at 74%. **(p. 990, Table 30–1)**

30.2   Numerous putative risk factors for the later expression of schizophrenia have been postulated and subjected to clinical investigation. Which of the following is true?

    A. First-degree relatives of schizophrenic patients have a 15%–20% risk of developing schizophrenia.
    B. Perinatal adverse events have been consistently associated with later development of schizophrenia; these events increase risk by 5%–10%, depending on the study.
    C. One compelling association between perinatal adverse events and the later expression of schizophrenia is the vulnerability of hippocampal pyramidal neurons to hypoxia.
    D. The association between winter birth and later development of schizophrenia is small and has not been consistently replicable.
    E. A monozygotic twin of a schizophrenia patient has a nearly 100% chance of developing schizophrenia, supporting a strong genetic component in the risk of this illness.

The correct response is option C.

Hippocampal pyramidal neurons are exquisitely sensitive to hypoxia.
    First-degree relatives of schizophrenic patients have a 3%–7% lifetime risk of manifesting schizophrenia, compared with 0.5%–1% in relatives of control subjects. The monozygotic twin of a person with schizophrenia has a 31%–78% chance of contracting the illness, compared with a 0%–28% chance for a dizygotic twin. Perinatal adverse events have been consistently associated with later

development of schizophrenia, although the overall risk of disease is only approximately 1%. The association between winter birth and later development of schizophrenia is small yet highly replicable. **(pp. 991–992)**

30.3   Anatomic and histopathological analyses have offered several compelling insights into the neuropathology of schizophrenia. Which of the following is true?

A. Magnetic resonance imaging (MRI) studies have revealed decreased volume of the superior temporal gyrus, and this finding has been correlated to the presence of delusions and negative symptoms.
B. In schizophrenic subjects, cells of the primary limbic structures have been found to have abnormal cell size and cell number but normal gross structure and area.
C. Basal ganglia enlargement (in the caudate nucleus and putamen) seen in schizophrenia is independent of treatment with antipsychotic medication.
D. The failure of normal neuronal migration during intrauterine development in schizophrenic patients is supported by the finding of excess neurons in lower, rather than superficial, layers of the cortex.
E. Decreased expression of glutamic acid decarboxylase (GAD) mRNA in schizophrenic patients is seen only with cell loss in the prefrontal cortex.

The correct response is option D.

During the second trimester of human fetal development, the failure of neurons to migrate upward from the ventricular wall to their target cortical layers has been evidenced by the finding of cortical neurons lower than expected.

MRI studies have revealed a volume decrease in the medial temporal cortical structures, hippocampus, amygdala, and parahippocampal gyrus and correlated it with the presence of hallucinations (Menon et al. 1995). In schizophrenic patients, abnormalities have been found in cell size, cell number, neuronal organization, and gross structure. Basal ganglia enlargement in schizophrenia occurs only after long-term treatment with neuroleptics. Decreased expression of GAD mRNA is found in the prefrontal cortex of schizophrenic patients without significant cell loss. **(pp. 992–994)**

30.4   Which of the following is true regarding neurotransmitters in schizophrenia?

A. The study of neurotransmitters and their metabolites in schizophrenia has greatly elucidated the neuropathology of this illness.
B. Dopamine type 2 (D_2)–family receptor density is increased in the caudate nucleus and putamen of schizophrenic subjects.
C. The recent finding of increased D_4 receptors in schizophrenic subjects is especially compelling in understanding the natural history of schizophrenia, because these receptors are unaffected by antipsychotic medication treatment.
D. Schizophrenic patients show an increased release of dopamine into the synapse during the chronic, but not acute, phases of their illness.
E. Norepinephrine levels are consistently and substantially elevated in schizophrenia, and noradrenergic antagonists decrease psychotic symptoms in these patients.

The correct response is option B.

D_2-family receptor density is increased in the caudate nucleus and putamen of schizophrenic patients (Cross et al. 1981).

The measurement of transmitters and metabolites has not critically contributed to the understanding of schizophrenia. Because D_4 density is known to increase with long-term neuroleptic treatment, further study is needed to draw final conclusions about the history of schizophrenia. Schizophrenic patients show an increased release of dopamine into the synapse during the acute phase of their illness. Norepinephrine levels have consistently been found to be elevated in schizophrenia, whereas noradrenergic antagonists do not reduce psychotic symptoms in schizophrenia. **(pp. 995–998)**

30.5 Several neuropsychological findings are reported in schizophrenia. Which of the following is true?

A. Identical twin studies have shown that the schizophrenic twin has poorer scores on intelligence, memory, and verbal fluency than the unaffected twin.

B. Likely because of the effects of paranoid cognitions, schizophrenic patients tend to perform well on instruments requiring sustained vigilance and attention.

C. First-degree relatives of schizophrenic patients exhibit a higher frequency of cognitive deficits but only when expressing psychotic symptoms.

D. Among relatives of schizophrenic subjects, the cognitive deficits are most dramatic in those with schizoid personality disorder.

E. The smooth-pursuit eye movement disorder in schizophrenia is only evident during active psychotic episodes.

The correct response is option A.

Studies of identical twins have shown that the schizophrenic twin performed significantly worse on assessments of intelligence, memory, attention, verbal fluency, and pattern recognition than the unaffected twin. Persons with schizophrenia consistently perform poorly on tasks that require sustained attention or vigilance. Several studies have observed that the first-degree relatives of schizophrenic patients demonstrate many of the cognitive deficits observed in schizophrenia, even though these individuals do not experience overt psychosis. The smooth-pursuit eye movement disorder in schizophrenia cannot be explained by disease-related factors or overt psychotic symptoms (Clementz and Sweeney 1990; Holzman 1987). **(pp. 999–1001)**

30.6 The impact of psychopharmacology on schizophrenia is an important clinical consideration. Which of the following is true?

A. There have been demonstrations of increased glucose metabolism in the caudate nucleus and putamen of schizophrenic patients after the administration of atypical antipsychotics, but this effect has not been seen with typical agents.

B. Dopamine agonists reduce dopamine synthesis by directly blocking the availability of precursor molecules.

C. The D_2 family of receptors (including D_2, D_3, and D_4) mediate the effects of antipsychotic agents, with most antipsychotics having activity at only one of these sites.

D. As a model for psychotic illness, ketamine is particularly illustrative because it induces both positive and negative symptoms.

E. Ketamine tends to induce psychotic symptoms idiosyncratic to the individual, which is unusual among psychotomimetic drugs.

The correct response is option E.

Ketamine tends to induce psychotic symptoms idiosyncratic to the individual, unlike psychotomimetics, which stimulate psychotomimetic symptoms typical of the drugs.

Increased glucose metabolism in the caudate nucleus and putamen of schizophrenic patients has been found following the administration of typical neuroleptics. Dopamine agonists reduce dopamine synthesis and release by their action at the dopamine autoreceptor. The D_2-family receptors mediate the antipsychotic actions of neuroleptics, with most neuroleptics having a measurable affinity at all three sites (D_2, D_3, and D_4). Ketamine stimulates the positive, not the negative, symptoms in schizophrenia. **(pp. 1006–1009)**

References

Clementz BA, Sweeney JA: Is eye movement dysfunction a biological marker for schizophrenia? a methodological review. Psychological Bulletin 108(1):77–92, 1990

Cross AJ, Crow TJ, Owen F: 3H-Flupenthixol binding in post-mortem brains of schizophrenics: evidence for a selective increase in dopamine D2 receptors. Psychopharmacology 74:122–124, 1981

Holzman PS: Recent studies of psychophysiology in schizophrenia. Schizophr Bull 13:49–75, 1987

Menon RR, Barta PE, Aylward EH, et al: Posterior superior temporal gyrus in schizophrenia: grey matter changes and clinical correlates. Schizophr Res 16:127–135, 1995

C H A P T E R   3 1

Neuropsychiatric Aspects of Mood and Affective Disorders

Select the single best response for each question.

31.1 Several neurochemical abnormalities have been implicated in the genesis and symptomatic expression of mood disorders. Which of the following is true?

    A. Consistent with a monoamine deficiency hypothesis, plasma norepinephrine is decreased in untreated depression.

    B. Acute antidepressant treatment increases norepinephrine turnover and neuronal norepinephrine uptake.

    C. A serotonin deficiency state in depression is supported by the finding of increased 5-hydroxytryptamine (serotonin) type 2 ($5\text{-}HT_2$) receptor binding in suicide victims.

    D. Acute treatment with antidepressants increases serotonin turnover and neuronal serotonin uptake.

    E. Cerebrospinal fluid (CSF) homovanillic acid and γ-aminobutyric acid (GABA) are both increased in untreated depression.

The correct response is option C.

A serotonin deficiency state in depression is supported by the finding of increased $5\text{-}HT_2$ receptor binding in the brains of suicide victims.

    Plasma norepinephrine is increased in patients with untreated depression. Acute antidepressant treatment decreases norepinephrine turnover and neuronal norepinephrine uptake. Acute treatment with antidepressants decreases neuronal serotonin uptake and serotonin turnover. CSF homovanillic acid and GABA are both decreased in patients with untreated depression. **(pp. 1023–1024)**

31.2 Various functional endocrine markers may have clinical implications in mood disorders. Which of the following is true regarding endocrine abnormalities in depression?

    A. The dexamethasone suppression test is abnormal in the vast majority of cases of depression.

    B. Depressed, euthyroid patients have nevertheless been shown to have elevated levels of circulating thyroid antibodies.

    C. Depressed patients have decreased corticotropin-releasing hormone (CRH) in the CSF.

    D. Corticotropin-releasing factor (CRF) binding in the frontal cortex of suicide victims is typically increased.

    E. Depressed patients show a prompt and large increase in thyroid-stimulating hormone (TSH) following administration of exogenous thyrotropin-releasing hormone (TRH).

The correct response is option B.

Depressed patients without overt thyroid dysfunction have nonetheless shown elevated levels of thyroid antibodies.

The dexamethasone suppression test, previously considered a marker of depressive illness, is abnormal in subsets of depressed patients. Depressed patients have increased CRH in the spinal fluid. CRF binding in the frontal cortex of suicide victims is typically decreased. Depressed patients show decreased blunted TSH response to exogenous TRH. **(p. 1025)**

31.3   Clinicians frequently encounter significant sleep complaints in depressed patients. Which of the following is true regarding the clinical and sleep laboratory findings in depressed patients?

A. Slow-wave sleep in increased in depression.
B. Reduced rapid-eye movement (REM) sleep latency is common in depression and is reversed by antidepressants.
C. Sleep deprivation produces greater antidepressant effects if administered in the first half of the sleep period.
D. Bipolar patients in a depressed episode also show predictable decreased REM latency.
E. In depression, the first REM period is of normal length and subsequent REM periods are lengthened.

The correct response is option B.

Reduced REM latency is the most reproducible sleep-related electroencephalographic finding in depressed patients, and this abnormality is reversed by most antidepressants (Sharpley and Cowen 1995).

Slow-wave sleep is decreased in depression. Sleep deprivation, particularly in the second half of the night, has an effect similar to medication. Bipolar patients who are hypersomnic do not show a consistent reduction in REM latency (Nofzinger et al. 1991). In depression, the first REM period is prolonged. **(pp. 1025–1026)**

31.4   Cognitive complaints and decrements in observed cognitive function are common in depression and may be the source of much of the patient's clinical suffering. Which of the following is true?

A. Impairment in language, perception, and spatial comprehension are common "primary" cognitive complaints in depression.
B. Depressed patients with cognitive complaints show similar degrees of functional impairment for both effortful and automatic cognitive tasks.
C. The pattern of specific memory deficits in depression simulates that seen in cortical, rather than subcortical, dementia.
D. Comparative studies in the cognitive status of treated patients show that tricyclic antidepressants (TCAs) and selective serotonin reuptake inhibitors (SSRIs) have similar effects on improving cognition.
E. The elderly patient with depressive pseudodementia may have an increased risk of eventual dementia, even if treatment responsive.

The correct response is option E.

The elderly patient with depressive dementia is at increased risk of subsequent dementia (King et al. 1995; Raskin 1986; van Reekum et al. 1999).

Impairment is most often encountered in the cognitive domains of attention, memory, and psychomotor speed. Studies show a differential impairment in effortful versus automatic cognitive tasks in depressed patients. The pattern of memory deficits in depression has been found to be statistically similar to that in subcortical dementia (Parkinson's and Huntington's diseases) in contrast to that in cortical dementia (Alzheimer's disease). Studies directly comparing TCAs with SSRIs have revealed improvements in memory for patients taking SSRIs but either no improvement or a worsening of cognition for those taking TCAs. **(pp. 1026–1028)**

31.5 Several neurologic conditions are associated with high risk for mood disorders and serve as convenient models for the study of neuroanatomic localization in depression. Which of the following is true?

A. Patients with traumatic brain injury show a high correlation between left-sided lesions and subsequent mood disorders.
B. Pathological emotions, both laughter and crying, are more common with left-sided lesions.
C. Positron emission tomography (PET) studies comparing unipolar depression, bipolar depression, and Parkinson's disease with depression have demonstrated that prefrontal, inferior parietal, and anterior cingulate gyrus hypometabolism are seen in all three types of depression.
D. Depression following lacunar subcortical stroke is associated with bilateral frontal lobe hypometabolism.
E. Because of the ongoing neuronal degeneration, Parkinson's disease with depression has decreased metabolism in the striatum.

The correct response is option C.

PET studies comparing unipolar depression, bipolar depression, and Parkinson's disease have demonstrated that prefrontal, inferior parietal, and anterior cingulate gyrus hypometabolism characterized the depressive syndrome, independent of underlying etiology.

Studies of patients with traumatic brain injury indicate a high correlation between mood disorders and right-hemisphere lesions (Grafman et al. 1986). Pathologic laughing is more common in patients with right lesions, whereas pathologic crying is seen in patients with left lesions. Depression following unilateral lacunar subcortical strokes is associated with temporal, rather than frontal, lobe hypometabolism. Parkinson's disease patients with depression have selective hypometabolism involving the caudate nucleus and prefrontal and orbitofrontal cortices (Jagust et al. 1992; Mayberg et al. 1990; Ring et al. 1994). **(pp. 1029–1032)**

31.6 Which of the following is true regarding functional neuroimaging in primary mood disorders?

A. Decreased frontal lobe function is the most robust finding in depression.
B. Although prefrontal activity is common in depression, it does not correlate directly with the degree of clinical symptoms.
C. Pretreatment hypometabolism in the rostral cingulate predicts response to antidepressant therapy.
D. Normalization of pretreatment frontal lobe hypometabolism is seen with TCAs and monoamine oxidase inhibitors (MAOIs) but not with SSRIs.
E. Likely because of the specificity of their effect on serotonin receptors, SSRIs result in downregulation of 5-HT_{2A} receptors, whereas TCAs do not.

The correct response is option A.

The most robust and consistent neuroimaging finding in depression is decreased frontal lobe function. Many studies have demonstrated an inverse relationship between prefrontal activity and depression severity. Pretreatment hypermetabolism in the rostral cingulate predicts response to antidepressant therapy, whereas hypometabolism does not. Normalization of frontal hypometabolism is seen with all antidepressants, including TCAs, MAOIs, and SSRIs. 5-HT_{2A} receptor downregulation has been demonstrated with SSRI and TCA treatment. **(pp. 1033–1035)**

References

Grafman J, Vance SC, Weingartner H, et al: The effects of lateralized frontal lesions on mood regulation. Brain 109:1127–1148, 1986

Jagust WJ, Reed BR, Martin EM, et al: Cognitive function and regional cerebral blood flow in Parkinson's disease. Brain 115:521–537, 1992

King DA, Cox C, Lyness JM, et al: Neuropsychological effects of depression and age in an elderly sample: a confirmatory study. Neuropsychology 9:399–408, 1995

Mayberg HS, Starkstein SE, Sadzot B, et al: Selective hypometabolism in the inferior frontal lobe in depressed patients with Parkinson's disease. Ann Neurol 28:57–64, 1990

Nofzinger EA, Thase ME, Reynolds CF, et al: Hypersomnia in bipolar depression: a comparison with narcolepsy using the multiple sleep latency test. Am J Psychiatry 148:1177–1181, 1991

Raskin A: Partialing out the effects of depression and age on cognitive functions: experimental data and methodological issues, in Handbook for Clinical Memory Assessment of Older Adults. Edited by Poon LW. Washington, DC, American Psychological Association, 1986, pp 244–256

Ring HA, Bench CJ, Trimble MR, et al: Depression in Parkinson's disease: a positron emission study. Br J Psychiatry 165:333–339, 1994

Sharpley AL, Cowen PJ: Effect of pharmacologic treatments on the sleep of depressed patients. Biol Psychiatry 37:85–98, 1995

van Reekum R, Simard M, Clarke D, et al: Late-life depression as a possible predictor of dementia: cross-sectional and short-term follow-up results. Am J Geriatr Psychiatry 7(2):151–159, 1999

C H A P T E R   3 2

Neuropsychiatric Aspects of Anxiety Disorders

Select the single best response for each question.

32.1 Various central nervous system (CNS) lesions and illnesses have been associated with anxiety symptoms and have thus served as models for certain anxiety disorders. Which of the following is true?

   A. Temporal lobe seizures, tumors, lobectomy, and arteriovenous malformations have been associated with panic attacks, with left-sided lesions showing a stronger association than right-sided lesions.
   B. Overlapping mechanisms between temporal lobe seizures have been proposed, but panic disorder is not associated with abnormal electroencephalogram (EEG) and does not respond to antiseizure medication.
   C. The striatal topography hypothesis of basal ganglia lesions held that putamen lesions led to tics, whereas caudate nucleus lesions led to obsessive-compulsive disorder (OCD) symptoms.
   D. Anxiety symptoms are a common neuropsychiatric prodrome in Huntington's disease and lead to generalized anxiety disorder (GAD), but not panic disorder or OCD.
   E. Anxiety symptoms in Alzheimer's disease are most common in the mild stages of illness (Mini-Mental State Exam [MMSE] score of 21–30).

The correct response is option C.

The striatal topography hypothesis of obsessions and compulsions states that caudate lesions are associated with OCD, whereas putamen lesions result in tics (Rauch and Baxter 1998).

   Temporal lobe seizures, tumors, arteriovenous malformation, lobectomy, and parahippocampal infarction have all been reported to present with panic attacks, particularly with right-sided lesions. Panic disorder may respond to anticonvulsants and is associated with abnormal EEG. In Huntington's disease, anxiety has been reported as the most common prodromal symptom, with later development of GAD, panic disorder, mixed anxiety and depression, or OCD. Anxiety symptoms in Alzheimer's disease patients are most common in the moderate stage of the illness. **(pp. 1050–1051)**

32.2 The common clinical syndromes of stroke and traumatic brain injury (TBI) are an important part of neuropsychiatric practice. In addition to the familiar mood and cognitive symptoms frequently seen in these conditions, anxiety disorders may also cause decreased patient function. Which of the following is true?

   A. Mixed anxiety and depression is more common with left-sided cortical stroke, whereas a "pure" anxiety disorder is more common after right-sided cortical stroke.
   B. Isolated worry is more common with right posterior cerebrovascular accident (CVA), whereas full-spectrum GAD is more common with right anterior CVA.
   C. Poststroke GAD is self-limited, even without treatment, and almost always resolves within 1 year.

D. Agoraphobia is much less common than GAD after stroke.

E. Posttraumatic stress disorder (PTSD) after TBI requires early, explicit memory of the traumatizing event.

The correct response is option A.

Anxiety with depression is associated with left cortical lesions, whereas anxiety alone is associated with right-hemisphere lesions. Worry is associated with anterior lesions and GAD with right posterior lesions. Astrom (1996) found a prevalence of 28% for GAD after stroke, with 19% continuing to have GAD at 3 years. Agoraphobia is even more common than GAD after stroke (Burvill et al. 1995). PTSD after TBI can develop even when the patient has neurogenic amnesia for the traumatic event. **(p. 1051)**

32.3 OCD is a fascinating and often disabling anxiety disorder that has strong neuroanatomical and neurophysiological implications. Which of the following is true?

A. Clinically effective treatment with a selective serotonin reuptake inhibitor (SSRI) leads to increased cerebrospinal fluid (CSF) 5-hydroxyindoleacetic acid (5-HIAA), suggesting adequate serotonin repletion.

B. Downregulation of serotonin terminal autoreceptors in orbitofrontal cortex follows successful treatment with SSRIs or electroconvulsive therapy (ECT).

C. OCD patients with tics are more likely to respond to SSRIs plus atypical, but not typical, antipsychotics.

D. Reduced caudate nucleus volume has been a consistent finding in OCD.

E. Cortico-striatal-thalamic-cortical (CSTC) activity normalization follows successful OCD treatment with medications or behavioral therapy.

The correct response is option E.

Baxter et al. (1992) reported that patients with OCD treated with either SSRIs or behavioral therapy had normalization of activity in CSTC circuits.

Treatment with SSRIs leads to decreased CSF 5-HIAA and a reduction of obsessive-compulsive symptoms. Downregulation of serotonin terminal autoreceptors in orbitofrontal cortex occurs only after relatively long periods and with high doses of medications and does not occur after ECT. OCD patients with tics are more likely to respond to augmentation of SSRIs with typical neuroleptics. An early study (Luxenberg et al. 1988) found reduced caudate volume in OCD patients, but not all subsequent research has replicated this finding. **(pp. 1053–1056)**

32.4 Panic disorder has also been subject to neuroanatomic and neurophysiological study. Which of the following is true?

A. The dorsal raphe nucleus sends serotonergic projections that stimulate the locus coeruleus.

B. The locus coeruleus sends noradrenergic projections that inhibit the dorsal raphe nucleus.

C. Fluoxetine has been shown to improve panic disorder symptoms; this improvement correlated with a simultaneous decline in a noradrenergic metabolite.

D. Basal ganglia functional abnormalities in panic disorder are as common as in OCD.

E. Panic disorder's clinical responsiveness to benzodiazepines correlates with increased peripheral benzodiazepine binding.

The correct response is option C.

Fluoxetine has been shown to improve panic disorder symptoms, with improvement correlated to the decline of 3-methoxy-4-hydroxy-phenylglycol (MHPG; a primary noradrenergic metabolite) in the plasma.

Serotonergic projections from the dorsal raphe nucleus generally inhibit the locus coeruleus, whereas projections from the locus coeruleus stimulate dorsal raphe nucleus serotonergic neurons. The basal ganglia have not commonly been implicated in panic disorder. Benzodiazepine receptor binding is decreased in panic disorder. (pp. 1056–1058)

32.5   Though often less dramatic in presentation than OCD or panic disorder, social phobia is a common source of clinical distress. Which of the following is true regarding the neuropsychiatry of social phobia?

   A. Although social phobia patients tend to have limited social lives, they are relatively unaffected educationally or vocationally.
   B. Enhanced cortisol response in social phobia has been found with fenfluramine, levodopa, and clonidine, suggesting multiple neurochemical pathways.
   C. Indirect evidence for a role of dopamine in social phobia includes an association of social phobia with Parkinson's disease and use of antipsychotic medications.
   D. Social phobia patients typically have abnormal responses on the dexamethasone suppression test, implicating a hypothalamic-pituitary- adrenal axis abnormality.
   E. Treatment of social phobia with SSRIs has been associated with reduced activity in the right temporal cortex.

The correct response is option C.

Social phobia may be associated with Parkinson's disease or may appear after the administration of neuroleptics (Stein 1998).

Patients with social phobia are more likely to be unmarried, to have weaker social networks, to fail to complete high school and college, and to be unemployed (Ballenger et al. 1998). Enhanced cortisol response in social phobia has been found only with fenfluramine and not with levodopa and clonidine. Social phobia patients have normal levels of urinary and plasma cortisol and normal dexamethasone suppression test results (Stein 1998). After treatment with SSRIs, patients with social phobia had significantly reduced activity in the left temporal cortex. (pp. 1060–1061)

References

Astrom M: Generalized anxiety disorder in stroke patients: a 3-year longitudinal study. Stroke 27:270–275, 1996

Ballenger JC, Davidson JR, Lecrubier Y, et al: Consensus statement on social anxiety disorder from the International Consensus Group on Depression and Anxiety. J Clin Psychiatry 59 (suppl 17):54–60, 1998

Baxter LR, Schwartz JM, Bergman KS: Caudate glucose metabolic rate changes with both drug and behavior therapy for OCD. Arch Gen Psychiatry 49:681–689, 1992

Burvill PW, Johnson GA, Jamrozik KD, et al: Anxiety disorders after stroke: results from the Perth Community Stroke Study. Br J Psychiatry 166:328–332, 1995

Luxenberg J, Swedo S, Flament M, et al: Neuroanatomical abnormalities in obsessive-compulsive disorder detected with quantitative X-ray computed tomography. Am J Psychiatry 145:1089–1093, 1988

Rauch SL, Baxter LR: Neuroimaging in obsessive-compulsive and related disorders, in Obsessive-Compulsive Disorders: Practical Management, 3rd Edition. Edited by Jenike MA, Baer L, Minichiello WE. St. Louis, MO, Mosby, 1998, pp 289–316

Stein MB: Neurobiological perspectives on social phobia: from affiliation to zoology. Biol Psychiatry 44:1277–1285, 1998

CHAPTER 33

Neuropsychiatric Disorders of Childhood and Adolescence

Select the single best response for each question.

33.1   Attention-deficit/hyperactivity disorder (ADHD) is a complex neuropsychiatric disorder with onset in childhood and with a variable persistence for years after diagnosis. In addition, neuropsychiatric comorbidity may complicate diagnosis and management. Which of the following is *not* true?

A. Conduct disorder is seen in 40%–70% of ADHD children.
B. ADHD is common in pediatric male patients with Tourette's syndrome.
C. The natural history of ADHD has been estimated to yield spontaneous remission in 30% by adolescence and up to 70% by adulthood.
D. Boys with ADHD have a stronger family history than do girls, particularly in male relatives.
E. Low birth weight, fetal alcohol exposure, and lead exposure are common etiological factors.

The correct response is option D.

Girls with ADHD have a stronger family history than do boys, suggesting even greater genetic loading but lower penetrance. **(pp. 1072–1073)**

33.2   An unusual but clinically significant side effect of antipsychotic treatment in children with Tourette's syndrome is

A. Secondary ADHD.
B. Phobic anxiety, leading to social phobia.
C. Major depression.
D. Neuroleptic malignant syndrome.
E. Paradoxical visual hallucinations.

The correct response is option B.

An unusual but significant side effect of neuroleptic treatment is the development of phobic anxiety, which can result in school avoidance and social phobias (Linet 1985; Mikkelsen et al. 1981). **(p. 1083)**

33.3 Down syndrome, or trisomy 21, is the most common chromosomal abnormality leading to mental retardation. Because of several central nervous system (CNS) and systemic anomalies, the life expectancy of these patients may be compromised. What is the average life expectancy in patients with Down syndrome?

A. 35 years.
B. 40 years.
C. 50 years.
D. 55 years.
E. 60 years.

The correct response is option C.

Life expectancy is approximately 50 years, with about 40% developing Alzheimer's disease by that point (Holland et al. 1998). **(p. 1085)**

33.4 Stereotypies are repetitive, apparently purposeless movements such as flicking, twirling, spinning of objects, hand flapping, whirling, and posturing. These movements are characteristic of which neuropsychiatric condition?

A. ADHD.
B. Tourette's syndrome.
C. Conduct disorder.
D. Autism.
E. Down syndrome with mental retardation.

The correct response is option D.

Stereotypies are common in autism, a rare but serious neuropsychiatric condition affecting 4–5 children per 10,000 births, with boys affected three to four times more often than girls. **(p. 1087)**

33.5 Seizure disorders are well known for their association with other neuropsychiatric comorbidity. A prominent association has been established between epilepsy, suicidality, and _____, which may be more prominent in temporal lobe epilepsy.

A. Manic episodes.
B. Catatonic posturing.
C. Hyperreligiosity.
D. Learning disabilities.
E. Self-destructive behavior.

The correct response is option E.

Self-destructive behavior. One of the earliest pioneering studies on the physiological determinants of suicide reported a strong positive association between paroxysmal electroencephalographic disturbances and suicidal ideation, attempts, and assaultive-destructive behavior (Struve et al. 1972). It has also been reported that the risk of completed suicide is four to five times greater in individuals with epilepsy than among patients without epilepsy and that this risk may be 25-fold greater in patients with temporal lobe epilepsy (Barraclough 1981; Mathews and Barabas 1981). **(pp. 1095–1096)**

33.6   Traumatic brain injury is the cause of more than 25% of hospital admissions in children and is a major source of persistent disability. Which of the following parameters of traumatic brain injury is most strongly related to clinical outcome?

A. Severity of brain injury.
B. Duration of posttraumatic amnesia.
C. Duration of coma.
D. Presence of brainstem injury.
E. Presence of increased intracranial pressure.

The correct response is option A.

Outcome is most strongly related to the severity of brain injury, although posttraumatic amnesia, length of coma, presence of brainstem injury, seizures, and increased intracranial pressure also affect prognosis (Beers 1992; Lieh-Lai et al. 1992). **(p. 1097)**

References

Barraclough B: Suicide and epilepsy, in Epilepsy and Psychiatry. Edited by Reynolds E, Trimble MR. New York, Churchill Livingstone, 1981, pp 72–76

Beers SR: Cognitive effects of mild head injury in children and adolescents. Neuropsychol Rev 3:281–320, 1992

Holland AJ, Hon J, Huppert FA, et al: Population-based study of the prevalence and presentation of dementia in adults with Down's syndrome. Br J Psychiatry 172:493–498, 1998

Lieh-Lai MW, Theodorou AA, Sarnaik AP, et al: Limitations of the Glasgow Coma Scale in predicting outcome in children with traumatic brain injury. J Pediatr 120:195–199, 1992

Linet LS: Tourette syndrome, pimozide, and school phobia: the neuroleptic separation anxiety syndrome. Am J Psychiatry 142:613–615, 1985

Mathews WS, Barabas G: Suicide and epilepsy: a review of the literature. Psychosomatics 22:515–524, 1981

Mikkelsen EJ, Detlor J, Cohen DJ: School avoidance and social phobia triggered by haloperidol in patients with Tourette's disorder. Am J Psychiatry 138:1572–1576, 1981

Struve FA, Klein DF, Saraf KR: Electroencephalographic correlates of suicide ideation and attempts. Arch Gen Psychiatry 27:363–365, 1972

C H A P T E R   3 4

Intracellular and Intercellular Principles of Pharmacotherapy for Neuropsychiatric Disorders

Select the single best response for each question.

34.1 Recent research has revealed the increasingly complex and critical roles of glial cells in neuronal function. Which of the following is true regarding this relationship?

A. Glial cells help maintain the critical balance between excitatory and inhibitory neurotransmitters by recapturing glutamate and γ-aminobutyric acid (GABA) from synapses and then returning them unaltered to their respective neurons.

B. Glutamate expresses excitotoxicity by the selective opening of sodium channels.

C. Glial cell line–derived neurotrophic factor (GDNF) has its specific trophic response only on dopamine neurons.

D. GDNF may ultimately represent a therapeutic intervention for Parkinson's disease and amyotrophic lateral sclerosis.

E. GDNF's high propensity to penetrate the blood-brain barrier is due to its structure as a short-chain peptide.

The correct response is option D.

GDNF has been proposed as a potential therapeutic agent for the treatment of Parkinson's disease, amyotrophic lateral sclerosis, and other neurodegenerative diseases.

Glial cells play a prominent role in recycling and conserving both glutamate and GABA by recapturing them from the synapse, converting them to glutamine and then returning glutamine to the presynaptic neurons for conversion back to the appropriate neurotransmitter (Shank et al. 1989). Prominent among glutamate's several cellular influences is the opening of specific calcium channels that allow the influx of calcium ions into neurons. The overstimulation of neurons via this mechanism has been associated with neurotoxicity and neuronal death. GDNF has been found to elicit a trophic response on several brain neuron types including motor neurons and noradrenergic, cholinergic, and serotonergic neurons (Bohn 1999). GDNF is a long-chain peptide and will not cross the blood-brain barrier. **(pp. 1124–1127)**

34.2 The mechanisms of neurotransmitter synthesis vary among the neurotransmitters that are involved in neuropsychiatric illnesses. Which of the following is true?

A. The final steps in the synthesis of neurotransmitters, including for neuropeptides, occur in regions proximate to the presynaptic storage site.
B. Proteins composing the presynaptic voltage-gated calcium channels are physically separated from the proteins devoted to storage vesicle docking and fusion.
C. Reserpine, as a model for presynaptic neurotransmitter storage disruption, produces a reversible effect on the storage of all biogenic amines.
D. Presynaptic $GABA_A$ and cholinergic receptors both operate by inducing hyperpolarization.
E. Presynaptic serotonin receptors, such as 5-hydroxytryptamine type 3 (5-HT_3), admit Ca^{2+} ions and produce depolarization.

The correct response is option E.

Presynaptic serotonin receptors, when activated, admit calcium into the neuron, thus promoting depolarization and neurotransmitter release (Ronde and Nichols 1998).

   The final synthesizing step for neuropeptides occurs within the neuronal soma. Neuropeptides must then be transported along the axon to the nerve terminal for storage. The proteins that compose the voltage-gated calcium channel are intimately bound to specific proteins associated with storage vesicle docking and fusion processes (Catterall 1999). Reserpine irreversibly destroys the ability of presynaptic storage vesicles to transport and store all biogenic amines (Krantz et al. 1999). Presynaptic cholinergic receptors admit calcium into the neuron when activated, thus promoting depolarization and neurotransmitter release (Ronde and Nichols 1998). **(pp. 1128–1129)**

34.3 Which of the following statements is true regarding the structure and function of postsynaptic receptors?

A. The most prevalent postsynaptic neuroreceptors form membrane channels or ionophores.
B. Receptors that act at allosteric sites, such as the benzodiazepine receptor, are typically coupled to G proteins.
C. Acetylcholine receptors include nicotinic and muscarinic; of these two types only the nicotinic involves actions of a G protein.
D. Long-term treatment with antidepressants has been shown to downregulate β-adrenergic receptors but not *N*-methyl-D-aspartate (NMDA) receptors in brain tissue.
E. Serotonin receptors operate via G proteins.

The correct response is option E.

Serotonin receptors operate via G proteins.

   The most prevalent postsynaptic neuroreceptors connect to a second-messenger system. Receptors that act at allosteric sites are typically coupled to GABA. Acetylcholine receptors include nicotinic and muscarinic subtypes, and only the muscarinic subtype involves actions of a G protein. Long-term treatment with antidepressants has been shown to downregulate β-adrenergic receptors and NMDA receptors in brain tissue. **(pp. 1133–1136)**

34.4   A drug has been shown to bind to a given postsynaptic receptor but then produce a physiological effect opposite to that produced by a natural neurotransmitter associated with that particular receptor class. This drug is thus acting as a(n)

A. Agonist.
B. Antagonist.
C. Inverse agonist.
D. Partial agonist.
E. Mixed agonist/antagonist.

The correct response is option C.

An inverse agonist is a drug that binds to a receptor but produces an effect opposite that of agonist activity.

A drug that binds to the receptor and causes a physiological response similar to that of a natural neurotransmitter is called an *agonist*. A drug that binds to the receptor and does not elicit a physiological response, but instead prevents agonists from binding to the receptor, is called an *antagonist*. Mixed agonist/antagonist drugs produce partial or limited agonist activities and may behave as antagonists in the presence of full agonists. **(p. 1134)**

34.5   Which of the following is true regarding the biochemical structure and/or function of postsynaptic G proteins and second messengers?

A. The G proteins are composed of numerous varieties of α, β, and γ subunits, all of which are interchangeable.
B. The α and γ subunits remain attached to each other and are the moiety that interacts with the neuroreceptor.
C. The action of lithium appears to be by blockade of inositol monophosphate.
D. Inositol triphosphate binds to receptors on the cell membrane and releases intracellular calcium.
E. G protein mechanisms are only seen for excitatory neurotransmitters.

The correct response is option C.

Lithium is well known to block inositol monophosphatase.

G proteins are composed of one each of three protein subunits termed α, β and γ, which are not interchangeable. Inositol triphosphate binds to a receptor on the endoplasmic reticulum. G protein mechanisms are linked to both inhibitory and excitatory receptors. **(pp. 1136–1139)**

34.6   The study of neurotransmitter/receptor mechanisms is of particular importance in evolving concepts of psychotic illness and in the development of more specific and less neurotoxic antipsychotic medications. Which is true regarding the atypical antipsychotic agents and their specific receptor binding properties?

A. Clozapine has a higher binding affinity for the dopamine D_4 receptor subtype than does haloperidol, accounting for its therapeutic efficacy.
B. The atypical antipsychotics have more 5-HT_{2A} binding affinity than do typical antipsychotics but not necessarily a higher binding affinity for 5-HT_{2A} than the D_2 dopamine receptor.
C. A specific D_4 antagonist was shown to be effective in the treatment of acute psychosis.
D. Haloperidol and atypical antipsychotic agents have similar binding affinity for 5-HT_6 and 5-HT_7 receptors.
E. Despite variations in their binding affinities for D_2 and 5-HT_{2A} receptors, the ratio of 5-HT_{2A} to D_2 binding affinities is similar for clozapine, olanzapine, and risperidone.

The correct response is option E.

The ratio of 5-HT$_{2A}$ to D$_2$ binding affinities is very close for clozapine, olanzapine, and risperidone, despite large variations in their individual binding affinities for D$_2$ and 5-HT$_{2A}$ receptors.

Clozapine has a lower binding affinity for the D$_4$ receptor than does haloperidol. Atypical antipsychotic drugs appear to have a higher binding affinity for 5-HT$_{2A}$ over dopamine D$_2$ receptors. A specific D$_4$ antagonist did not demonstrate efficacy for treating acute psychosis. Haloperidol and atypical antipsychotics such as clozapine, olanzapine, and risperidone have quite different affinities for 5-HT$_6$ and 5-HT$_7$ receptors. **(pp. 1141–1142)**

References

Bohn MC: A commentary on glial cell line-derived neurotrophic factor (GDNF). From a glial secreted molecule to gene therapy. Biochem Pharmacol 57:135–142, 1999

Catterall WA: Interactions of presynaptic Ca2+ channels and snare proteins in neurotransmitter release, in Molecular and Functional Diversity of Ion Channels and Receptors. Edited by Rudy B, Seeburg P. New York, New York Academy of Sciences, 1999, pp 144–159

Krantz DE, Chaudhry FA, Edwards RH: Neurotransmitter transporters, in Neurotransmitter Release. Edited by Bellen HJ. Oxford, UK, Oxford University Press, 1999, pp 145–207

Ronde P, Nichols RA: High calcium permeability of serotonin 5-HT3 receptors on presynaptic nerve terminals from rat striatum. J Neurochem 70:1094–1103, 1998

Shank RP, William JB, Charles WA: Glutamine and 2-oxoglutarate as metabolic precursors of the transmitter pools of glutamate and GABA: correlation of regional uptake by rat brain synaptosomes. Neurochem Res 16:29–34, 1989

Psychopharmacologic Treatments for Patients With Neuropsychiatric Disorders

Select the single best response for each question.

35.1 The general approach to psychopharmacology in neuropsychiatric patients is subject to certain clinical caveats, owing to the implications of neurologic illness on the metabolism and end-organ effects of psychopharmacological agents. Which of the following is true?

A. A poststroke patient with depression and aggression should be treated preferentially with tricyclic antidepressant monotherapy.

B. A brain-injured patient with complex partial seizures comorbid with manic symptoms of labile affect and impulsive behavior should first receive combination therapy with lithium and phenytoin to maximize control of each symptom domain.

C. Because of the increased sensitivity of neuropsychiatric patients to side effects with psychotropic medications, initial and ultimate or final doses should be less than those for other adult patients.

D. Because of the likelihood of cognitive impairment and compliance problems, the psychiatrist should rely on medication blood levels as a marker for medication efficacy.

E. Treatment of psychiatric symptoms before they exacerbate the patient's neurological illness may improve overall functioning (e.g., in multiple sclerosis).

The correct response is option E.

Early treatment of a psychiatric symptom before it can exacerbate the neurologic disorder may significantly improve the patient's overall functioning (i.e., emotional distress has been shown to worsen or precipitate exacerbations of multiple sclerosis) (Grant et al. 1989).

A poststroke patient with depression and aggression should be preferentially treated with SSRIs. A brain-injured patient with complex partial seizures and labile affect and impulsivity should be treated with carbamazepine or valproate rather than with phenytoin and lithium combined. Patients with central nervous system (CNS) pathology should be started at a lower dose of medication and titrated more slowly, although in the end they may ultimately require the same dose of medication as the nonneurologic patient. Medication blood levels do not necessarily correlate with medication efficacy but may give information about compliance and drug metabolism. **(pp. 1153–1155)**

35.2 For clinical purposes, it is useful in neuropsychiatry to group depression, apathy, and deficit states. Which of the following is true regarding these conditions?

A. The use of relatively activating antidepressants should be avoided in anxiously depressed neuropsychiatric patients.
B. Apathy states refer to cognitive and behavioral slowing due to a mood disorder.
C. There is a consistent relationship among many neuropsychiatric illnesses that depression severity predicts more rapid subsequent neurological deterioration and ultimately disability.
D. Postmortem studies of depressed patients with Alzheimer's disease have shown deficits in both the serotonin and norepinephrine pathways.
E. Systemic medications, such as corticosteroids, calcium-channel blockers, and β-blockers, are consistently shown to induce depression when mean differences in treated versus untreated groups are examined.

The correct response is option D.

Postmortem studies of depressed patients with Alzheimer's disease have shown deficits in the serotonin and norepinephrine pathways.

It has not been proven that the use of activating antidepressants in anxious depressed individuals should be avoided. Apathy states refer to cognitive and behavioral slowing that occurs in the absence of mood disturbance (Levy et al. 1998). Most studies have failed to find a consistent association of severity of depression with progression of neurologic illness or subsequent disability and have failed to show group mean differences between treated and untreated patients for systemic medications. **(pp. 1155–1157)**

35.3 Which of the following is true regarding the treatment of depression in neuropsychiatric patients?

A. Selective serotonin reuptake inhibitors (SSRIs) have a role both in post–cerebrovascular accident depression and in pathological crying in the absence of full-spectrum depression.
B. Tricyclic antidepressants (TCAs) are as well-tolerated as SSRIs in patients with multiple sclerosis.
C. A major benefit of SSRIs in neuropsychiatric patients is the absence of risk of extrapyramidal side effects (EPS).
D. Bupropion is problematic in neuropsychiatric patients because its propensity to induce seizures is idiosyncratic rather than dose dependent.
E. Methylphenidate may induce euphoric mood in patients with Parkinson's disease.

The correct response is option A.

SSRIs have been found useful in the treatment of emotional incontinence (i.e., pathologic crying in the absence of depression).

In patients with multiple sclerosis, TCAs produced twice the side-effect rate of SSRIs (Scott et al. 1996). EPS are the most common CNS side effects with SSRIs. Bupropion has the potential to lower seizure threshold; however the dose dependence of this side effect may make lower doses more acceptable. Patients with Parkinson's disease experience no euphoria in response to methylphenidate. **(p. 1158)**

35.4   Which of the following is true regarding the treatment of depression, apathy, and deficit states in neuropsychiatric illness?

   A. Psychostimulants must be used with caution in patients with brain injury because of a propensity to increase seizure frequency.
   B. Pemoline has been shown to effectively treat fatigue in patients with multiple sclerosis and has been well-tolerated.
   C. Electroconvulsive therapy (ECT) has not been effective in depression due to Huntington's disease because of ECT-induced worsening of movement disorder symptoms.
   D. Parenteral benzodiazepines are a highly effective alternative to ECT in catatonic states.
   E. Catatonia is more likely to be caused by psychotic states than affective disorders.

The correct response is option D.

Parenteral benzodiazepines are a highly effective alternative to ECT in catatonic states.
   Psychostimulants tend to reduce seizure frequency in brain injury patients. Pemoline has been shown to treat fatigue in 50% of multiple sclerosis patients, although the drug is not well tolerated because of anorexia, irritability, and insomnia. ECT is an effective treatment in Huntington's disease patients. Catatonia is more strongly related to affective illness than to psychosis. **(p. 1159)**

35.5   Which of the following is true regarding psychosis in the context of neuropsychiatric illness?

   A. Psychosis is common in patients who have had a stroke and who have multiple sclerosis.
   B. Psychosis in human immunodeficiency virus (HIV) dementia, as opposed to Alzheimer's disease, is strongly associated with severe dementia and malignant disease progression.
   C. Psychosis in Parkinson's disease is caused by the degeneration of cortical structures and is not a side effect of antiparkinsonian medications.
   D. Clozapine has been documented as the most effective antipsychotic agent in Parkinson's disease, and low doses are often effective.
   E. In dementia, risperidone 2 mg/day has been demonstrated to have a low risk of EPS.

The correct response is option D.

The only medication with confirmed antipsychotic benefit that does not worsen Parkinson's disease is clozapine, with a mean dose of 25 mg.
   Psychosis is relatively uncommon in stroke and multiple sclerosis. In Alzheimer's disease, psychosis is associated with more severe dementia and rapid disease progression than in HIV dementia. Antiparkinsonian drugs are a common cause of psychosis in Parkinson's disease patients. In dementia-related psychosis, risperidone 2 mg/day has been demonstrated to have rates of EPS ranging between 32% and 50%. **(pp. 1163–1165)**

35.6   Which of the following is true regarding mania and anxiety in neuropsychiatric illness?

A.   Mania in patients with traumatic brain injury is no more common than in the general population.
B.   Patients with multiple sclerosis are more likely to have mania than are populations of general psychiatric inpatients.
C.   Agitation is as common in multi-infarct vascular dementia as in Alzheimer's disease.
D.   Anxious states are common in damage to the right anterior inferior temporal lobe, whereas manic states are less localized.
E.   Serotonergic deficiencies in Alzheimer's disease have been consistently related to behavioral agitation.

The correct response is option B.

Patients with multiple sclerosis are more likely to have mania than both general and psychiatric inpatient populations.

There is much greater incidence of mania in patients with traumatic brain injury than in the general population. There is a high incidence of agitation in Alzheimer's disease but not in multi-infarct dementia. Both anxious and manic states are common with damage to the right anterior inferior temporal lobe. Serotonergic deficiencies in Alzheimer's disease have been inconsistently related to agitation (Mintzer et al. 1998). **(pp. 1166–1169)**

35.7   β-Blockers may be a relatively underutilized group of medications for agitated states in neuropsychiatry. Which of the following is true?

A.   Placebo-controlled studies show a greater than 50% rate of response.
B.   Response is typically manifest within 3 weeks.
C.   Anti-agitation effects are due to central, rather than peripheral, effects.
D.   Secondary depression induced by β-blockers is relatively common and leads to discontinuation of treatment.
E.   The dose of propranolol may need to be as high as 800 mg/day, although lower doses are typical.

The correct response is option E.

The dose of propranolol may need to be titrated up to 800 mg/day, although doses in the range of 160–320 mg/day have been effective. Placebo-controlled studies of β-blockers show a modest (30%) rate of response. Response may take up to 8 weeks, and both central and peripheral effects may contribute to therapeutic action. Secondary depression due to β-blockers appears to be a rare occurrence, but these medications are contraindicated in patients with asthma, chronic obstructive pulmonary disease (COPD), insulin-dependent diabetes, congestive heart failure, angina, and hyperthyroidism (Yudofsky et al. 1987). **(p. 1176)**

References

Grant I, Brown GW, Harris T, et al: Severely threatening events and marked life difficulties preceding onset or exacerbation of multiple sclerosis. J Neurol Neurosurg Psychiatry 52:8–13, 1989

Levy ML, Cummings JL, Fairbanks LA, et al: Apathy is not depression. J Neuropsychiatry Clin Neurosci 10:314–319, 1998

Mintzer J, Brawman-Mintzer O, Mirski DF, et al: Fenfluramine challenge test as a marker of serotonin activity in patients with Alzheimer's dementia and agitation. Biol Psychiatry 44:918–921, 1998

Scott TF, Allen D, Price TRP, et al: Characterization of major depression symptoms in multiple sclerosis patients. J Neuropsychiatry Clin Neurosci 8:318–323, 1996

Yudofsky SC, Silver JM, Schneider SE: Pharmacologic treatment of aggression. Psychiatric Annals 17:397–407, 1987

CHAPTER   3   6

Psychotherapy for Patients With Neuropsychiatric Disorders

Select the single best response for each question.

36.1   Psychological defense mechanisms are best conceptualized as existing on a continuum from the most mature (representing the highest level of psychological health), through an intermediate group of less mature, to the most immature (typifying psychotic functioning). Which of the following defenses is classified among the most mature defenses?

A. Suppression.
B. Reaction formation.
C. Rationalization.
D. Displacement.
E. Isolation.

The correct response is option A.

The most mature defenses are sublimation, suppression, and laughter. Less mature are reaction formation, rationalization, displacement, and isolation. The most immature are denial, splitting, merging, projection, and projective identification. **(p. 1200)**

36.2   There have been described a number of misidentification syndromes that may result from neuropsychiatric illness that are manifest in specific patterns of perception and behavior. If a patient perceives that a previously familiar person has now assumed another bodily form, the phenomenon is referred to as

A. Capgras's delusion.
B. Frégoli type misidentification.
C. Metamorphosis.
D. Subjective doubles.
E. Reverse Frégoli type misidentification.

The correct response is option B.

In the Frégoli type misidentification, a patient perceives that a familiar person has assumed another bodily form.

In Capgras's delusion, people are perceived as being replaced by identical doubles. In intermetamorphosis, the perception is that both minds and bodies of people are interchanging. In subjective doubles of the Capgras's type, the patient perceives that unseen doubles, phantom boarders, or deceased persons are felt to be present. In the autoscopic type of subjective doubles, a person's own double is projected onto another person in the positive form, and in the negative form, the person cannot see himself or herself, even in a mirror. In reverse subjective doubles, the person feels either like an impostor or as if in the process of being replaced. In the reverse Frégoli type, the person believes that other people are misidentifying him or her as if he or she has Frégoli delusions of misidentification. (pp. 1200–1201)

36.3   Psychological functioning in patients with schizophrenia has been offered as an explanatory model for the understanding of psychological functioning of patients with other neuropsychiatric illnesses. All of the following psychological processes are shared between schizophrenic patients and those with neuropsychiatric illnesses *except*

A. Catastrophic reactions to overwhelming stress.
B. Involuntary concreteness.
C. Incapability of moving among different levels of abstraction.
D. Fear of novelty.
E. The use of emotions to overcome cognitive problems.

The correct response is option E.

In most neurologic patients, emotions are used to overcome cognitive and linguistic problems, whereas in schizophrenic patients, emotions are used to compensate for poor command of affects. (p. 1202)

36.4   Which of the following is true of the psychological functioning of patients with traumatic brain injury?

A. The patient's family is most disrupted by the patient's cognitive difficulties rather than emotional symptoms.
B. Psychotherapeutic interventions should be delayed until the emergency of irritable temper, typically at 3 months after injury.
C. To avoid burnout of treatment team staff, day-long one-on-one rehabilitation is best avoided.
D. Problem-solving exercises should begin with the concrete and, after mastery, should then proceed to the more abstract.
E. Posttraumatic headache rarely persists beyond 3 months and thus is unlikely to disrupt psychotherapy at this point.

The correct response is option D.

Problem-solving exercises should move from the concrete to the abstract.

   The family of the patient with traumatic brain injury is more affected by the disruption of emotions and object relations than the patient's cognitive difficulties. Psychotherapeutic interventions should begin soon after the patient is hospitalized because management of the emotions is crucial to recovery. Childs (1985) recommends one-on-one work all day with the patients. Posttraumatic headache persists for 6 months in up to 44% of patients, thus exerting a significant negative effect on therapy. (p. 1204)

36.5   Intervention with the patient's family aids in greater functional recovery following traumatic brain injury. Which of the following is true?

A. Family involvement should begin only after a strong therapeutic alliance with the patient has been established over time.
B. The psychotherapist should avoid informing the family in great detail about the process of functional recovery, so as to preserve patient privacy.

C. Family members should be warned about the possibility of being manipulated by the injured patient.

D. The therapist should avoid a stance of active advocacy for the brain-injured patient in the family situation.

E. The therapist should guard against the family generalizing the patient's learning to novel situations, focusing instead on the issue at hand only.

The correct response is option C.

Family members of patients with traumatic brain injury should be warned about the possibility of being manipulated by the patient.

The family should be integrated into the treatment process from the beginning. The therapist should be highly directive, informed, and informing; be an advocate for the patient; and assist generalization of learning from one situation to another. **(p. 1209)**

36.6 The neuropsychiatrist may be called upon to treat the unfortunate victim of paralyzing spinal cord injury. Which of the following is true regarding the psychological and psychotherapeutic aspects of spinal cord injury?

A. Clinically significant major depression is seen in the majority of patients within 6 months of injury.

B. Cognitive-behavioral interventions for spinal cord injury patients have been associated with fewer readmissions and higher levels of adjustment.

C. An internal locus of control predicts depression 2 years after injury.

D. Because of the high risk of depression, cognitive-behavioral therapy should routinely be offered to all victims of spinal cord injury.

E. Because of the demographics of those affected by spinal cord injury, individual and group psychotherapy should focus on introspection and avoid action orientation.

The correct response is option B.

Persons who received cognitive-behavioral therapy had fewer readmissions and higher levels of adjustment.

Manifest depression is not an inevitable psychological sequel to spinal cord injury. Bodenhamer et al. (1983) found that patients with spinal cord injuries reported less depression and more anxiety and optimism than their caregivers predicted. An external locus of control was associated with depressive mood 2 years after admission. Not everyone with spinal cord injury needs cognitive-behavioral therapy, but those with reported high levels of depressive mood benefited greatly. Demographically, these patients are young men who are activity oriented and may resist group or individual therapy that is not action oriented and peer involving. **(pp. 1211–1212)**

36.7 Parkinson's disease is a neurodegenerative disorder with notable psychiatric comorbidity. Which of the following is true regarding the psychotherapeutic issues involved in Parkinson's disease?

A. To assist the patient's process of acceptance of his or her illness, early use of support groups (including more advanced patients) is advised.

B. Behavioral interventions for parkinsonian gait include focus on straightening posture, attention to balance, and renormalizing the arm swing.

C. The psychotherapist must be attuned to the presence of violent and threatening hallucinosis in 30% of patients treated with L-dopa.

D. Greater degrees of gait disturbance, tremor, and postural abnormalities reliably predict cognitive impairment.

E. As with other neurodegenerative diseases, communication in Parkinson's disease is compromised by language impairments.

The correct response is option B.

Behavioral interventions for patients with Parkinson's disease are aimed at standing straighter, balancing better, starting more quickly to walk, and stepping more rhythmically with normal arm swings.

Patients in the early stages of Parkinson's disease should be exposed as little as possible to patients in the most advanced stages in support groups or waiting areas. Hallucinosis occurs in 30% of patients treated with L-dopa, but the hallucinations are nonthreatening and can be managed without neuroleptics. Bradykinesia and rigidity, but not tremor, gait disturbance, or posture, predict cognitive impairment. Parkinson's disease is distinct from other neuropsychiatric disorders because of the paucity of language impairment. **(pp. 1219–1221)**

36.8   Multiple sclerosis is another major chronic illness of the central nervous system that will come to the attention of the psychiatrist. Which of the following is true of the psychological and psychotherapeutic aspects of multiple sclerosis?

A. Paradoxical serenity (pleasant affect despite neurologic impairments) is more common early in the illness.

B. The chronic and unpredictable nature of multiple sclerosis may lead to excess dependence on physicians.

C. Despite the possibility of functional losses of frontal lobe function, the patient should be challenged to undertake significant reordering of defenses when symptomatic.

D. The psychotherapist should limit theoretical and practical approaches to supportive psychotherapy models only.

E. Dementia in multiple sclerosis affects memory encoding and storage more than retrieval.

The correct response is option B.

Multiple sclerosis may lead to patients' excessive dependence on physicians.

Paradoxical serenity is more frequent later in the course of the disease. When involvement of the frontal lobe is present in multiple sclerosis, it is important not to attempt sweeping revision of defenses. The psychotherapist should apply a spectrum of strategies, from insight-oriented to supportive, in a flexible way as determined by the patient's needs. Dementia in multiple sclerosis affects retrieval more than encoding and storage of information. **(pp. 1226–1228)**

References

Childs AH: Brain injury: "now what shall we do?" problems in treating brain injuries. Psychiatric Times, April 1985, pp 15–17

Bodenhamer E, Achterberg-Lawlis J, Kevorkian G, et al: Staff and patient perceptions of the psychosocial concerns of spinal cord injured persons. American Journal of Physical Medicine 62:182–193, 1983

C H A P T E R   3 7

Cognitive Rehabilitation and Behavior Therapy for Patients With Neuropsychiatric Disorders

Select the single best response for each question.

37.1   The general approach of the clinician to the cognitive rehabilitation of the neuropsychiatric patient establishes the therapeutic context of the clinical goals. Which of the following is true?

   A. In cognitive rehabilitation after stroke, reorganization of motor skills is possible for only the first year after the stroke.
   B. Cognitive rehabilitation of the traumatic brain injured patient is likely to focus on a specific cognitive deficit rather than general approaches to memory and attentional disturbances.
   C. Because of cognitive deficits, anger management training is unlikely to benefit the traumatic brain injury patient.
   D. Psychostimulant medication may facilitate rehabilitation in patients with frontal lobe injuries.
   E. Psychological recovery in traumatic brain injury is usually greater for ecologically relevant behaviors than on performance on standardized tests.

The correct response is option D.

The treatment of frontal lobe injury with dopaminergic agents may beneficially affect other rehabilitation efforts (Kraus and Maki 1997). In cognitive rehabilitation after stroke, brain reorganization for motor skills may be possible even a decade past the time of the stroke (Liepert et al. 2000). A treatment program designed primarily to treat patients with head injury is likely to focus on the amelioration of attentional and memory deficits, whereas one designed for stroke patients is likely to focus on a more specific deficit, such as language disorder. Anger management training has been shown to benefit the traumatic brain injury patient. Psychological recovery in traumatic brain injury shows larger effects as measured by standardized tests than as measured by ecologically relevant behaviors (Ho and Bennett 1997). **(pp. 1238–1239)**

37.2   Several instrumental models using computers to facilitate cognitive rehabilitation have been developed. Which of the following is *not* an area of training in the Orientation Remedial model of Ben-Yishay and associates (Ben-Yishay and Diller 1981)?

   A. Attending and reacting to environmental signals.
   B. Timing responses to changing environmental cues.
   C. Practice of active vigilance.
   D. Time estimation.
   E. Synchronization of response to simple, repetitive rhythms.

The correct response is option E.

The Orientation Remedial program developed by Ben-Yishay and associates consists of five separate tasks that are presented by microcomputer and vary in difficulty. The tasks involve training in the following areas: 1) attending and reacting to environmental signals, 2) timing responses in relation to changing environmental cues, 3) being actively vigilant, 4) estimating time, and 5) synchronizing of response with complex rhythms. **(p. 1239)**

37.3   A cognitively impaired patient is instructed to enhance his or her memory function by constructing a story from newly presented material to facilitate encoding. This is an example of

    A. Semantic elaboration.
    B. Face-name association.
    C. Peg mnemonics.
    D. Method of loci.
    E. Direct retraining.

The correct response is option A.

Semantic elaboration involves constructing a story out of new information to be remembered.

    Face-name association involves associating the components of the name with a distinctive visual image. *Peg mnemonics* requires the patient to learn a list of peg words and to associate these words with a given visual image. *Method of loci* involves the association of verbal information to be remembered with locations that are familiar to the patient. **(pp. 1239–1240)**

37.4   Which of the following is true regarding visual-perceptual disorders and the approaches to cognitive rehabilitation?

    A. Visual-perceptual deficits are most common after left-sided occipital stroke.
    B. Hemispatial neglect syndrome is most often experienced in the right hemispace.
    C. A light board with colored lights and a fixed target is used for visual scanning training.
    D. Visual scanning training as a sole cognitive intervention was found to improve visual-perceptual functioning in brain-injured patients when compared with those patients who were treated with standard occupational therapy.
    E. Hemispatial neglect is most common in right-hemisphere stroke.

The correct response is option E.

Hemispatial neglect is most common in right-hemisphere stroke.

    Deficits in visual perception are most common in patients who have undergone right-hemisphere cerebrovascular accidents (Gouvier et al. 1986). Hemispatial neglect syndrome is characterized by the inability to recognize stimuli in the contralateral visual field. Visual scanning training, with addition of other tasks, was found to improve visual-perceptual functioning in a group of patients with brain injury in comparison with a group of similar patients who received standard occupational therapy (Gordon et al. 1985). A light board with 20 colored lights and a target that can be moved is used for visual scanning training. **(p. 1241)**

37.5   There may be spatial localization of neuropsychiatric symptoms following injury to the cortex that affects the cognitive rehabilitation of patients. Which of the following behavioral symptoms is more commonly a sequel of temporal, rather than frontal, lobe injury?

    A. Paranoid ideation.
    B. Social disinhibition.

C. Reduced attention.
D. Distractibility.
E. Affective lability.

The correct response is option A.

Individuals with temporal lobe dysfunction can show heightened interpersonal sensitivity, which can evolve into frank paranoid ideation. Frontal lobe dysfunction secondary to stroke or tumor shows social disinhibition, reduced attention, distractibility, impaired judgment, affective lability, and more pervasive mood disorder. **(pp. 1243–1244)**

37.6   In a behavioral treatment paradigm, the behavioral therapist has noted a reliable relationship between a specific target behavior and an environmental consequence. The therapist removes the environmental consequence, and the target behavior thereafter is reduced to a near-zero rate of occurrence. This phenomenon is called

A. Positive reinforcement.
B. Negative reinforcement.
C. Punishment.
D. Antecedent.
E. Extinction.

The correct response is option E.

Extinction occurs when the reliable relation between a specific behavior and an environmental consequence is removed, thus reducing the target behavior to a near-zero rate of occurrence.

A behavior followed by an environmental consequence that increases the likelihood that the behavior will occur again is called a *positive reinforcer*. A behavior followed by the removal of a negative environmental condition is called a *negative reinforcer*. A behavior followed by an aversive environmental event is termed a *punishment*. When behavior is controlled or affected by the events that precede it, these events are called *antecedents*. **(p. 1245)**

References

Ben-Yishay Y, Diller L: Rehabilitation of cognitive and perceptual deficits in people with traumatic brain damage. Int J Rehabil Res 4:208–210, 1981

Gordon W, Hibbard M, Egelko S, et al: Perceptual remediation in patients with right brain damage: a comprehensive program. Arch Phys Med Rehabil 66:353–359, 1985

Gouvier WD, Webster JS, Blanton PD: Cognitive retraining with brain damaged patients, in The Neuropsychology Handbook: Behavioral and Clinical Perspectives. Edited by Wedding D, Horton AM, Webster J. New York, Springer, 1986, pp 278–324

Ho MR, Bennett TL: Efficacy of neuropsychological rehabilitation of mild-moderate traumatic brain injury. Archives of Clinical Neuropsychology 12:1–11, 1997

Kraus MF, Maki M: Effect of amantadine hydrochloride on symptoms of frontal lobe dysfunction in brain injury: case studies and review. J Neuropsychiatry Clin Neurosci 9:222–230, 1997

Liepert J, Bauder H, Miltner WHR, et al: Treatment-induced cortical reorganization after stroke in humans. Stroke 31(6):1210–1216, 2000

CHAPTER 38

Ethical and Legal Issues in Neuropsychiatry

Select the single best response for each question.

38.1 The legal concept of *competency* has a substantial impact on neuropsychiatric practice, particularly in those patients presenting with cognitive impairments. Which of the following is true?

A. The definition, requirements, and application of the term *competency* vary widely, depending on the issue at hand.

B. Capacity refers to an individual's abilities with regard to display of intact cognitive and decision-making function in a wide range of acts.

C. A mentally ill patient can be held to be incompetent based entirely on the evaluation of a clinician.

D. Institutionalization for mental illness results in the patient being assumed to be incompetent.

E. All minors are assumed to be incompetent.

The correct response is option A.

The definition, requirements, and application of competency vary widely, depending on the circumstance in which it is being measured.

Capacity refers to an individual's actual ability to understand or to form an intention with regard to some act. A patient with a neuropsychiatric disorder that produces mental incapacity generally must be declared incompetent judicially before his or her legal rights can be abridged. The person's current or past history of physical or mental illness is but one factor to be weighed in determining whether a particular test of competency is met. Lack of capacity or competency cannot be presumed either from treatment for mental illness or from institutionalization. In some situations, minors are assumed to be incompetent. However, there are exceptions to the general rule, such as minors who are considered emancipated, mature, or competent to consent in some cases of medical need or emergency. (pp. 1258–1259)

38.2 The neuropsychiatrist may be called upon to comment on a patient's ability to give informed consent for or to refuse a proposed medical/surgical procedure. All of the following standards apply to this determination *except*

A. Communication of a choice.

B. Demonstration of understanding of information provided.

C. Appreciation one's current situation and the relative risks and benefits of treatment options.

D. Absence of a cognitive disorder on standardized examination.

E. Rationality in the decision-making process.

The correct response is option D.

The absence of a cognitive disorder on standardized examination is not a standard applied for determining incompetency in decision making. **(p. 1260)**

38.3 When the patient is deficient in the capacity to make medical decisions, a proxy decision maker may be needed. There are several alternatives provided for in the law. Which of the following surrogate choices may be excluded from decisions regarding the treatment of mental disorders?

A. Court-appointed guardian.
B. Treatment review panel.
C. Substituted consent of the court.
D. Institutional administrator or committee.
E. Proxy consent of next of kin.

The correct response is option E.

Proxy consent of next of kin may be excluded for treatment of mental disorders. **(p. 1261, Table 38–2)**

38.4 The "right to die" may lead to psychiatric evaluation and need for opinion. Which is true regarding the legal status of this issue?

A. The *Cruzan* decision held that the state did not have the right to maintain the patient's life against the family's wishes.
B. The Court distinguished between food and water on the one hand and mechanical ventilation on the other.
C. Physicians are now strongly encouraged to seek clear and competent instructions regarding future treatment decisions, such as with a living will.
D. The right to decline life-sustaining treatment is absolute.
E. As a result of the *Cruzan* decision, physicians will not be held liable for overtreatment of critically ill patients.

The correct response is option C.

When treating severely or terminally impaired patients, physicians must seek clear and competent instructions regarding foreseeable treatment decisions, in the form of a living will or durable power of attorney agreement.

The *Cruzan* decision held that the state of Missouri had the right to maintain the patient's life, even to the exclusion of the family's wishes. The Court did not distinguish between food and water and other life-sustaining mechanical measures. The right to decline life-sustaining treatment is not absolute. Liability may arise from overtreating critically or terminally ill patients just as much as for stopping life-sustaining treatment. **(pp. 1261–1262)**

38.5 Which is true regarding the insanity defense in criminal proceedings?

A. This defense requires that the accused is incompetent to stand trial.
B. The insanity defense is estimated to be successful in only 10% of the times it is attempted.
C. The estimated rate of not guilty by reason of insanity is estimated at less than 1% of all felony arrests.
D. The Comprehensive Crime Control Act of 1984 supports the volitional prong of the insanity defense.
E. Mental retardation is not an adequate basis for the insanity defense; only Axis I illnesses are allowed.

The correct response is option C.

The annual average of not guilty by reason of insanity verdicts is well below 1% of all felony arrests (Melton et al. 1997). Defendants with mental disabilities who are found competent to stand trial may seek acquittal on the basis that because of the insanity, they were not criminally responsible for their actions at the time the offense was committed. The insanity defense is successful in only one out of four times it is attempted. The Comprehensive Crime Control Act of 1984 eliminates the volitional or irresistible impulse prong of the insanity defense. Mental retardation may represent an adequate basis for an insanity defense under certain circumstances. **(pp. 1267–1268)**

Reference

Melton GB, Petrilla J, Poythress NG, et al: Psychological Evaluations for the Courts, 2nd Edition. New York, Guilford, 1997

CHAPTER 39

Educational and Certification Issues in Neuropsychiatry

Select the single best response for each question.

39.1 The requirement for clinical experience in neurology in psychiatry residency programs in the United States has been specified by the Accreditation Council on Graduate Medical Education (ACGME) since 1987. How many months of neurology experience are presently required?

A. 1 month.
B. 2 months.
C. 3 months.
D. 4 months.
E. 6 months.

The correct response is option B.

The ACGME requires that general psychiatry residency training include a minimum of 2 months of neurology experience. **(p. 1289)**

39.2 The 2001 revision of ACGME Essentials for Training in General Psychiatry includes all of the following requirements *except*

A. Diagnosis and treatment of neurologic disorders encountered in psychiatric practice.
B. Indications for and limitations of common neuropsychological tests.
C. Systemic instruction in neurobiology.
D. Performance and recording of neurological examination.
E. Interpretation of electroencephalograms (EEGs).

The correct response is option E.

The 2001 revision of ACGME Essentials for Training in General Psychiatry does not require interpretation of EEGs. **(p. 1291)**

39.3 Combined training in psychiatry and neurology has been proposed as an educational pathway for neuropsychiatrists. Which of the following is true?

A. Combined training requires a minimum of 5 years.
B. The first postgraduate year requires 6 months of internal medicine and 3 months each of neurology and psychiatry.
C. A minimum of 2 years must be spent each in psychiatry and neurology.
D. All U.S. combined residencies are currently accredited.
E. Dual training leads to dual board eligibility and dual hospital privileges.

The correct response is option E.

Dual training leads to dual board certification and dual hospital privileges. Combined neurology and psychiatry training requires a minimum of 6 years, including 8 months of internal medicine during the internship year. Two and one-half years must be spent each in psychiatry and neurology. As of 1999, 9 of the 16 combined neurology and psychiatry residencies were accredited. **(p. 1303)**